MW01287212

Advance Praise for *Psychologically Sound*

"As we try to understand President Trump as a human being and his motivations, Dr. Roth, in this beautifully written psychobiography, presents an alternative view to the pathological diagnoses ascribed to him by many mental health professionals. Reaching below the surface of the words and actions of this 'chaos' President, Dr. Roth comes up with a different 'persona' that humanizes the man. *Psychologically Sound* will elicit much controversy and discussion in our politically supercharged environment."

—Steven S. Sharfstein, M.D.,
President Emeritus, Sheppard Pratt Health System

"*Psychologically Sound: The Mind of Donald J. Trump* is a remarkable work. It is the first description of Donald Trump that really conveys the totality and depth dimensions of the nature of the man. It is warm, empathic, and respectful not only to the President, but also to the reader. Roth is able to convey the President as a gifted, driven, complicated, and in some ways flawed person, but more importantly, a real human being. It is also well written, clear, and free of political bias.

"This is a must read for those who really want a more balanced picture and a deeper understanding of what drives our President."

—Robert L. Pyles, M.D., Past-President,
American Psychoanalytic Association

"Dr. Roth has beautifully applied the tools of modern psychology to provide the first in-depth and balanced understanding of the astonishing and fascinating Donald J. Trump. Supporters and detractors alike will learn the full human story of a man who, for all his tweets, has been a baffling puzzle to many and deeply understood by few."

—Stephen Rittenberg, M.D.
Former Editor,
Journal of Clinical Psychoanalysis
Medical Director (Retired),
The Treatment Center of The New York
Psychoanalytic Institute and Society

THE MIND
OF
DONALD J. TRUMP

PSYCHOLOGICALLY SOUND

SHELDON ROTH, M.D.

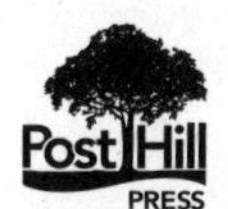

A BOMBARDIER BOOKS BOOK
An Imprint of Post Hill Press
ISBN: 978-1-64293-329-1
ISBN (eBook): 978-1-64293-330-7

Psychologically Sound:
The Mind of Donald J. Trump

Cover Design by Cody Corcoran

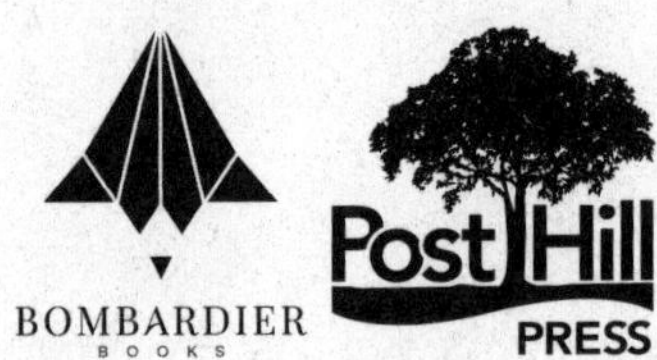

Post Hill Press
New York • Nashville
posthillpress.com

Published in the United States of America

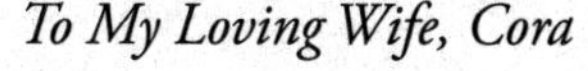

To My Loving Wife, Cora

CONTENTS

INTRODUCTION

Psychologically Sound draws on my five decades of psychiatric and academic experience to demonstrate the soundness and humanness of President Donald J. Trump's mind through a long life richly overflowing with people, events, and challenges. Creating a holistic view that avoids a misleading focus on Trump as businessman, celebrity, or politician frees us to see Trump as a complete person whose life fits together, reflects a sound mind, and is recognizably human. Yet, *Psychologically Sound* does not shy away from the unbearable. Trump is depicted in active mental struggle as opposed to mindless repetition, as human as anyone, and yet, mysteriously, so different from the rest of us, one person leading 330 million people. Understanding how President Trump is more like the rest of us than otherwise increases our capacity to bear the mysterious, and maybe also, each other.

In pursuit of grasping lifelong holistic themes, and unique to *Psychologically Sound,* is a psychological dream analysis of Trump's musings on his favorite film, *Citizen Kane.* This dream analysis, "Citizen Trump," reaches into Trump's early family life, his businesses, and his two failed marriages as well as his long relationship with Melania Trump. Among many reader surprises will be the discovery of how Trump values love and marriage above wealth as a core ingredient in a happy life. After his second divorce and prior to his marriage to Melania, he said, "I feel guiltiest about not having had a successful marriage.... [My parents] were married sixty-three years.... The part of my life I think I'm most disappointed in is that I have not had the great marriage.... I come from a home where marriage was incredible." And in reference to *Citizen Kane*, he noted, "In Kane you learn that wealth is not everything. He had the wealth but he didn't have the happiness." "Citizen Trump" establishes the values of love, marriage, and family as bedrock elements of Trump's character.

Similarly, the media's neglect of the immense importance of Reverend Norman Vincent Peale on Trump's worldview and speaking style is truly astounding. One needs a whole spiritual picture of Donald Trump to glimpse the ever-present influence of Reverend Peale. Trump awards the title of "mentor" to only two people in his life: his father Fred C. Trump Sr. and Reverend Peale. Trump states, "Dr. Peale...was perhaps the greatest speaker I have ever watched.... I would leave that church feeling like I could listen to another three sermons." In Dr. Peale's writings we can hear Trump. For example, Peale says, "Never think of yourself as failing.... So always picture "success" no matter how badly things seem to be going at the moment.... Stand up to an obstacle. Just stand up to it, that's all, and don't give way under it, and it will finally break. Something has to break, and it won't be you, it will be the obstacle.... Every problem has in it the seeds of its own solution. If you don't have any problems, you don't get any seeds." This last positive Pealeism is woven into Trump's accounts of his successes in real estate. The chaos of real estate that appealed to Trump as one of Peale's "problem" opportunities and its relevance for the current White House chaos is explored as well as Trump's ease of fabrication, especially on the campaign trail (which never ends for Trump), as it unlocks his speaking style—"affective rhetoric is effective rhetoric."

It will also surprise people that Trump is not only familiar with the Swiss psychiatrist and psychoanalyst Carl G. Jung, but leans on Jung as a guide and clarifier of his own psychology. "[Jung] keeps my mind open to my unconscious.... [Jung] will fine-tune your intuitions and instincts.... You will gain a technique for seeing into—versus reading into—the people around you.... Jung will give you insights into yourself and the ways in which you and other people operate.... Each of us has a persona. We need it for survival. It's the face we put on for public use." The failure of Trump's first two marriages, as well as the near twenty-two-year relationship with Melania Trump, are explained through Trump's understanding of the tension between one's "persona" and one's "private self." Fiercely independent, yet dependently embedded in his personal social fabric, particularly his family and a few closely held friends, Trump has attempted a balance between a branded persona and a more hidden private self. In part, this conflict has kept his virtues less visible. Uncovering the dichotomy of persona versus private self, reveals Trump as distinctly thoughtful and introspective, a capacity rarely depicted, if ever, in the general media.

To capture a sense of a person requires appreciation of what that person has experienced in life, what the moment reflects of the past and even what it hints of the future. So, the themes of this book swirl back and forth through threads of Trump's life, present and past, while also gathering up those around him. For example, misogyny. What of misogyny? Long before it was politically correct, culturally chic, or legally and culturally mandated, Trump, with little fanfare, was a champion of women. Especially in business, Trump's open pathway for professional advancement benefited women. Trump's promotion of women, unfettered by cultural convention, or macho real estate practices, flies in the face of frequent accusations of rampant misogyny. For example, building Trump Tower, against all advice (including his "mentor" father's), Trump hired the first female construction manager in New York real estate history, and to this day, the majority of executive positions in the Trump Organization are held by women with pay equal to men. How Trump's pro-women attitude has continued and played out in the White House is explored as well as tracing the fascinating family roots of Trump's openness to women's professional abilities through an analysis of four generations of formidable Trump women. These four generations reflect a deep psychological orientation for Donald J. Trump: "The Wall of Family." This familial castle is a separate social empire, it supersedes all other social relationships, encompasses "loyalty," and interestingly, also leads to one of President Trump's handicaps in The White House—no one reaches the level of trust he has in family. One thread of personality's fabric inevitably joins others, and only then is a person recognizable and appreciated.

Psychologically Sound builds a picture of an individual enmeshed in the world, and enmeshed with a consistency of personality, beliefs, and quests—all with a sound mind. Sound, except with one major exception—the period following the demoralizing failure of his marriage to Ivana Trump. I describe this special period of regressive turmoil as also one of diminished business acumen, the time of financial fiascos in gambling casinos (the bankruptcies), and faulty social skills resulting in the unhappiest and shortest marriage of the three—Marla Maples. The variations of these three marriages reveal the depth and complexity of Trump. These are not simple marital repetitions; they are each revealed as strikingly unique.

And, although soundness of mind may not be of question in certain of President Trump's actions, their dubious nature or value leaves me with many misgivings about Trump. I invite readers to share my struggles with those misgivings while still maintaining support of our president. As stated earlier, "this book does not shy away from the unbearable." I imagine many readers are faced with a similar challenge, and will find it helpful to see that "misgivings" are realistic, likely quite variable since "all politics is local," but do not necessarily eliminate firm support of Trump.

Anyone interested in this book has a special question in mind: "Is President Trump fit to be president?" What is fitness for the presidency? American history has answers, intriguing answers, but all inevitably lead to further questions. I use two concepts, comparing transactional and transformational goals of leaders, with special attention to the power of persuasion in relation to achieving those goals. Trump is presented as a transformational leader with a handicapped, excessive reliance on single-handed communication as a primary tool of persuasion. Extremely important in this perspective is a discussion of the riotous circus of pathological psychiatric diagnoses applied to

President Trump. These pathological diagnoses are unequivocally refuted. Sadly, and painfully, psychiatric science can be abused by partisan politics. With great puzzled pleasure, regarding presidential fitness, I share with readers an illuminating page from American history that reveals President Trump's similarities to President James K. Polk, "The Mendacious," reviled as the worst American president in history in the nineteenth century and now included among the "greats." History is the ultimate judge.

In considering President Trump's life, beyond soundness of mind, is awe. I would lack sufficient motivation to write this book without consideration of the concept of awe. Awe connotes a mysterious mixture of comprehension and incomprehension, reverence, respect, wonder, astonishment, and on its edges, fear. From a small band of ex-colonists to a burgeoning power of 330 million people, our psychology seeks a supreme leader—for America, fortunately modulated by the checks-and-balances crafted by our revolutionary founders—a single person out of a sea of people is entrusted with leadership. The mantle of the presidency, in and of itself, evokes awe. The nature of Trump's sweeping, proposed generational changes—transformational—is essential to this emotional package. *Psychologically Sound* wrestles with nature, nurture, and fate, and their shaping one person, Donald Trump—of sound mind and recognizably human—to be the vehicle of change for many millions, but we are still left with mystery, and for some of us, that mystery includes awe.

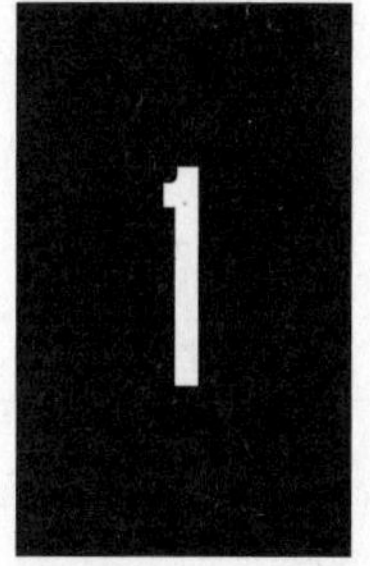

CITIZEN TRUMP

Citizen Kane

Cinema offers a rich repository of human life, both real and imagined. Although the theater's blank screen is projected on with an endless kaleidoscope of images, how we see them depends on who we are. We can find others and ourselves in images and stories that capture our imagination. Our favorite films occupy a special place in our minds and hearts; such films capture enduring values and clues as to how we live or long to live. Orson Welles's 1941 cinematic masterpiece *Citizen Kane* is President Donald J. Trump's favorite film. *Citizen Kane* was nominated for nine Academy Awards, including Best Picture, and won the Oscar for Best Original Screenplay. Interestingly enough, Trump's favorite film does wonders to help us understand his own character.

The Film's Tale

Charles Foster Kane, the film's central character, lives through the late nineteenth century and first half of the twentieth century. In childhood he acquires great wealth through his mother's chance acquisition of a mining fortune. The wealth causes his mother to send him far away into the care of the mine's lawyer for proper education and elite breeding. Kane's mining wealth increases phenomenally, and demonstrating extraordinary business skill, he builds a vast publishing empire. Specializing in yellow journalism, idiosyncratically single minded and rebellious, Kane makes and creates the news. Headline lies become reality for his readers. Before CNN, Trump learned about "fake news" from *Citizen Kane*. Handsome, a spellbinding speaker, eager for power, and a financial tycoon, he enters politics. With eyes on the White House, he is on the verge of a landslide victory as Governor of New York when a sex scandal crushes his campaign and destroys his first marriage.

Thumbing his nose at society, Kane marries his singer mistress, builds an opera house for her, but fails to make her an opera star. She is a talentless, unmotivated victim of Kane's overblown ambition. Ever imperious, Kane retreats to a vast, seaside, Hearst-like castle in Florida called Xanadu (named from Samuel Taylor Coleridge's poem *Kubla Khan*).

His opulent fortress is filled with endless European art, statues, and valuable collections. His wife, tortured by Kane's inability to love and feeling like one of his collectibles, ultimately leaves him. Isolated, bitter, surrounded by an army of servants, he dies alone, and on his deathbed, utters a last word, "Rosebud." The film's narrative is Kane's reconstructed life seen through the eyes of a journalist as he searches for the meaning of "Rosebud." While he never does, the cinematic audience is let in on the secret.

Journalists and Donald J. Trump

The elusive mystery of Rosebud for the film's journalist, which he felt would explain the essentials of Charles Foster Kane's psychology, is both fascinating and ironic. President Trump's current heated feud with journalists hinges on how blind they are to the facts about him and are purveyors of "fake news." But there was a time in New York when Donald Trump thrived on the adoration of journalists; their enthusiasm for him was described in a New York Times magazine article as akin to "rock star fans." Everyday New Yorkers felt a similar keenness. Walking down the street people approached Trump and touched him, hoping his good fortune would rub off on them (Geist, 1984). In wooing his second wife, Marla Maples, Trump often sent her glowing press clippings about himself, a rather happy and unique form of journalistic endorsement of one's love life.

A. J. Benza is a highly successful, male version of the late Hedda Hopper (the queen of newspaper tattlers of the 1940s and '50s). In 2016, Benza shared his journalistic memories of Donald Trump:

> *In the late '80s and '90s, it was impossible NOT to write about Donald. He was everywhere. And he was doing everything. He was getting divorced from Ivana, marrying Marla, becoming a dad again, fixing up Wollman's Rink, renovating 40 Wall Street or Trump Place. It got to a point, wherever I felt I HAD to be for the good of the column, I'd run into him. SpyBar—check, a quick bite at Bowery Bar—check. Knick's playoff games—check. Front row at Victoria Secret's fashion show—check. So, I'd write the column and not including him felt like I wasn't doing my job.... For years...Donald was a guy who lived and died in the columns.... I once said, he doesn't check his pulse in the morning—he checks the papers to see if he's alive.... Trump's honesty (yes, I said it) was always refreshing. And a lot of people are seeing that today. He says things many of us feel. Sure, he puts his foot in his mouth sometimes (Friedersdorf, 2016).*

Judge Jeanine Pirro shared similar observations in her 2018 book, *Liars, Leakers and Liberals*:

> *Believe it or not, there was a time when the media adored Donald Trump. Throughout the 1980s and '90s, you could hardly pass a newsstand without seeing Donald's face on the covers of glossy tabloids and fifty-cent newspapers. There were stories about*

> *him gallivanting around New York and attending charity galas, photographs of him standing in front of new buildings, and long stories about business in which he'd give tips to aspiring entrepreneurs. Whether it was about renovating a dilapidated hotel into a showpiece, erecting soaring towers that drew the envy of his peers or, mostly out of his own pocket, building a skating rink in Central Park, the media reported positive news about Donald Trump on a very regular basis.... [Pirro describes Trump's constant use of the telephone] ... aside from his friends and business partners, the people who called most often were newspaper and magazine reporters. He always took their calls, too. Reporters couldn't get enough of Donald Trump. He was funny and engaging, and his quotes always sold newspapers, magazines, and ad space on news shows.... Even when the press was taking shots at Donald's lavish lifestyle, there was respect for him. Occasionally, the press would even publish the acts of charity that Trump preferred to keep secret. Donald tipped waiters, doormen, workers, and everyone.*

Notably, during those heady New York years when Donald J. Trump was a special darling of the daily newspaper gossip columns he played a cat-and-mouse game with those journalists. He often telephoned gossip columnists in a disguised voice, identifying himself as Donald Trump's non-existent publicist

John Barron (Trump confessed to an obsession with the name Barron, a name he later gave to his youngest son, and John is his own middle name). In these "anonymous" interchanges he proffered tidbits of Donald Trump gossip, some true, and others a bit stretched. As the source of "quasi-fake news," perhaps the proverbial shoe was once on the other foot. President Trump's enmeshed tangle of ambivalent symbiosis with the media goes back a long way. It seems fitting that a frustrated journalist is at the center of Trump's favorite film, and that its central character, Charles Foster Kane, leverages the political power wealth can enable as a newspaper publisher.

Imagine the artistic awe Orson Welles might reap contemplating President Donald J. Trump's fascination with *Citizen Kane.* Welles's cinematic mirror of art held up to nature contained a past, a present, and perhaps a prophecy—with some major differences.

Trump Analyzes Citizen Kane

In 2002, Errol Morris, a critically acclaimed documentarian, was requested by the Academy of Motion Picture Arts and Sciences (The Oscars) to film various celebrities discussing their favorite movie. Donald Trump was one, choosing *Citizen Kane,* and his remarks are revealing (Canfield, 2016). Since the film is fantasy, despite Kane's similarities to publishing magnate William Randolph Hearst, there was, in fact, no real Charles Foster Kane. Trump's interest in *Citizen Kane*, and what he finds most powerful in its impact on him, helps us to understand what is important in life for him.

Rosebud

Trump suggests that "Rosebud" is the single "most significant word" in cinema history and is the key to understanding the meaning of *Citizen Kane*. "Rosebud" (Attention! Spoiler alert!) is the trade name on the sled a young Kane is playing with in the Colorado snow when his mother abruptly announces to him that that very moment he is going away with the mine's lawyer, Thatcher, a man the boy had never met before. The child is reduced to helpless rage and grief. At the film's conclusion a cleaning crew is throwing unvalued Xanadu trash into a gigantic burning fireplace. As the camera pans into the eliminating inferno, we see the childhood sled, its time-encrusted veneer melting, revealing the name "Rosebud."

"Rosebud," says Trump, "brings a lonely sad figure back into his childhood." In a deft manner, Trump tuned into the childhood sadness of the grown-up Kane and knew, intuitively, it was a lifelong sadness. Trump's precise empathy finds the heart of the matter and can only come from a person who knows it firsthand, has thought about it, and has come to grips with it. "Rosebud" brought Kane back to a period of life that was secure, innocent, happy, and to the best of his knowledge, loving, until he was suddenly cast out. Grief stricken, he raged against leaving his mother.

At age thirteen, Donald Trump was abruptly shipped off to The New York Military Academy at Croton-on-the-Hudson in upper New York State. From early elementary school, his father, Fred C. Trump Sr., was troubled with the Queens, New York, Kew-Forest school due to complaints of Donald's rebellious infractions and lack of discipline. But what tipped Fred C. Trump Sr. over was discovering that, over a long period, Donald had been secretly going into Manhattan on Saturdays with his close friend Peter Brant. Just over the East River, a short subway ride away, Manhattan was a land of exotic adventure compared to quiet Queens. The two boys roamed the streets, Central Park, and ogled the tawdry mysteries of Times Square. This uncontrolled adventuring in dangerous, tempting Manhattan, raised great concern in Fred C. Trump Sr. Sending his son to military school was an attempt to bring greater discipline and safety to his life. Bear in mind that about twelve years later, against his father's urgent business warnings, Donald Trump moved to Manhattan to build a real estate empire. Donald Trump easily empathized with young Kane's emotional pain as he was abruptly torn from the home nest. But, unlike Kane, Trump found ways to integrate family, love, and work. I elaborate on this merger in later chapters.

One also must wonder about the age at which Fred C. Trump Sr. sent his son away (thirteen). Fred C. Trump Sr. was just five months shy of his thirteenth birthday when his German-born father, Frederich, died in the 1918 pandemic flu. President Trump's oldest sister, retired Judge Maryanne Trump Barry, has said of their father: "My father's father died when he was a teenager, and Dad went to work to support his mother and two siblings as a carpenter and as a builder's mule, hauling carts of lumber to construction sites when it was too icy for the mules to climb the hills" (Katz, 2016). Fred's German father, Frederich, was actually eleven when his father died in 1877, but similar to Donald, Frederich was sent away at fourteen as an apprentice barber in a distant city. Three generations of Trump males were challenged to prove themselves in early adolescence. We might speculate that this shared challenge at a developmentally malleable age built into them a conviction that adversity is not only to be expected in life, but it presents an optimal setting for mastery. Donald Trump often expresses this attitude in his view that chaos offers opportunity, or as his mentor, Reverend Norman Vincent Peale, aphorized: "Every problem has in it the seeds of its own solution. If you don't have any problems, you don't get any seeds" (Peale, 1952). This proposition will be later elaborated on in a discussion of Reverend Norman Vincent Peale's influence on President Trump.

Love and Marriage

Hidden within a useful nocturnal dream are a dreamer's central, unresolved, gnawing conflict and a solution; the pathway to understanding is often guided by a powerful dream image (Roth, 1987). Similarly, with psychological intuitiveness, Trump fathoms that the solution to Kane's grief and failed love lies in unlocking the mysteries of "Rosebud" and its links. Kane's two marriages failed, and that is why when Morris asks Trump what advice he would give Kane if he had such an opportunity, Trump unhesitatingly says, "Get yourself a different woman." Trump, like Kane, had two failed marriages. "Get yourself another woman," is not the flip rejoinder of a thoughtless serial husband. It is the remark of a man intent on finding permanent love with a woman, such lasting love being a primary goal in life.

In 1999, prior to marrying Melania and after the divorce from his second wife, Marla, on *Good Morning America*, Diane Sawyer asked Donald Trump, "What do you feel guiltiest about?" He replied:

"I feel guiltiest about not having had a successful marriage, because coming from parents that were married sixty-three years, and having gone through all that, I think that is the thing I would probably feel most guilty about. My business has been unbelievable, so I can't feel guilty about business. I think I've done well; I've made a lot of people very proud...very rich. But the business thing has been pure. The part of my life I think I'm most disappointed in is that I have not had the great marriage. And I would have thought that would have happened.... Some of my friends get divorced, but their parents were divorced twice or three times. I come from a home where marriage was just incredible...my parents truly loved each other."

Trump has outlined the mistakes of his first two marriages (more on this important topic later). With Melania as his third marriage, Trump feels an equilibrium he could not find with Ivana and Marla. About those two marriages, in an eerie similarity to Kane, Trump has said, "I create stars...I love creating stars...I've done that with Ivana...I've done that with Marla... unfortunately, after they are a star, the fun is over for me. It's like a creating process. It's almost like creating a building. It's pretty sad.... They [were] completely different from each other.... Ivana is a tough and practical businesswoman; Marla is a performer and actress.... I have come to realize these two exceptional women represent the extremes of my personality" (Trump and Bohner, 1997). This self-reflection distinguishes

Trump from Kane who handled conflict solely with action and no understanding. Seemingly avoiding his extremes, Donald fell in love with Melania who had fashioned a self-made, successful modeling career before meeting him. Melania did not require Donald to make her a "star." In many ways Melania more resembles Trump's mother than did either of his first two wives, or, for that matter, any other romantic relationship of the past. A later discussion of Mary Anne MacLeod Trump, Trump's mother, will make those similarities more apparent. From the point of view of love, Donald Trump has come home.

In contrast to his earlier marriages, Donald's relationship with Melania resembles that of his parents. Much of Melania and Donald's life in Trump Tower was dictated by domestic routine. Donald Trump worked long hours like his father who returned home late in the day, had dinner with his wife, and then continued to work at home. At Trump Tower, after work, Donald, by elevator, would ascend to their apartment, and have a quiet dinner together, relieved that she was distant from his business concerns. Then, peacefully, they often engaged in separate activities. Sometimes Melania might join him in watching TV (often sports). Even when he was single, Donald often ended a hectic and sophisticated business day with a walk to a local Korean grocery store to buy a bag of chips, which was immediately taken back to his bedroom at Trump Tower, available for dinner and TV munching. Like Mary MacLeod's comfort with Fred Trump's domestic isolation, Melania gives comfortable room for the same isolating trait in Donald.

President Trump and First Lady Melania occupying separate bedrooms in the White House has raised eyebrows, but the couple had the same arrangement at Trump Tower for many years. Without equivalent media dismay, President John F. Kennedy and Jacqueline Kennedy Onassis had the same nocturnal arrangement. Along with Trump's adhesive attachment to public attention is a counterbalancing desire for isolation. Trump's current early hour of the day retreat to the White House bedroom is very similar to his behavior in Trump Tower; a blitz of daytime activity in the office was followed by protective isolation in his bedroom.

The media laments the relative unavailability of Melania for traditional First Lady interviews, desiring access to her intimate thoughts and feelings. During her recent trip to Africa (in October 2018), a photo of Melania in front of Egypt's Sphinx—an ancient mystery and a modern one—struck me as wondrous photographic synchronicity. The First Lady responded to interview questions graciously, but sparingly, and to the point (Rogers, 2018). In her natural, sequestered stance, Melania reflects the private, unavailable-to-the-press self of Donald. Trump—the private self. This protected face of Trump is explored in Chapter Three, "The Persona and the Person." As a side note, outside of the family, Trump's mother, Mary, was often characterized as "tight lipped." One could not use the same characterization for either Ivana Trump or Marla Maples, both press-worthy loquacious.

Like many marriages, as time passes, the underlying psychological similarities of the partners are increasingly revealed.

Donald Trump has described how quiet Melania Trump is compared to his first two wives, and his older children have referred to her as "the portrait" (Kranish and Fisher, 2016). Yet he can depend on her for a strong, clear opinion when asked. Indeed, Melania speaks five languages: English, Italian, French, German, and Slovenian. Her sphinx-like persona belies deft mental acuity. Melania Trump has said, "We give ourselves and each other space. I allowed him to do [what he wants], to have his passion and dreams come true, and he let me do the same. I believe [in] not changing anybody. You need to understand [another person] and let them be who they are" (Kranish and Fisher, 2016).

For almost thirty years, Donald Trump has intermittently investigated a presidential run. Trump's beyond twenty-year relationship with Melania, which includes eleven years of marriage, potentially contributed to a level of familial security—enabling him to take the final step. In subsequent chapters we will continue to explore their relationship, and the possible impact of recent revelations of alleged extramarital affairs by Trump (Borchers, 2018).

Love and Loss

A capacity to love and bear loss are perhaps the two most important emotional tasks of life. And, they are linked. Love sustains an ability to bear loss. In the simplest example, stepping outside one's earliest home, losing one's parents and family becomes bearable as we find other loves and other homes, be they people or purpose. Finding love is usually preceded by loss. It is commonplace for people to find their first meaningful love in high school or college; both are connected to saying "goodbye" to home. Finding new love is a re-finding.

So, I am impressed that Trump's focus on the important elements of *Citizen Kane* centers on just that. He does not suggest that wealth brings happiness. Of Kane's enormous wealth he observed that "In Kane you learn that wealth is not everything. He had the wealth but he didn't have the happiness.... Wealth does in fact isolate you from other people...a protective mechanism [develops].... You have your guard up more than if you don't have wealth. The fall was not financial; it was a personal fall, but a fall nonetheless." Interestingly, Kane's Xanadu, so incredibly similar to Trump's Mar-a-Largo, is not seen by Trump as an answer to Kane's bitter unhappiness.

The Lesson of *Citizen Kane*

Like a dream that offers a turbulent dreamer a solution, Trump uncovers a solution for Kane: "Find yourself a different woman." Trump interprets Kane's unresolved sadness as resulting from a failure in love, and perhaps can feel that sadness with a sense of "there but for the grace of God (or love) go I." Without a loving relationship, Kane's life unraveled. We shall see how something similar happened to Donald Trump as his loving marriage to Ivana fell apart, and marriage to Marla did not repair that loss. From Trump's vantage point, the screen-fantasy-dream of *Citizen Kane* is viewed as a lesson on "how-to-not-do-it" and learns for himself what is needed "to-do-it." Kane's childhood loss may be similar to Trump's, but they're not identical. Kane's mother effectively abandoned her child, and the coldness of that relationship is reflected in Kane's inability to love or care for others.

Trump reveres his childhood and his parents. His father was very attached to him and regularly visited him at military school. There is no evidence of discord between Donald and his father over the decision to send him to military school. In fact, even when Donald's father was in his nineties, with significant dementia and confusion over recognizing family names, one name he never had difficulty with was "Donald" (Barstow, Craig, and Buettner, 2018). Trump developed significant real estate with his father while in college, and afterward worked alongside him for five years in Brooklyn and Queens before embarking to Manhattan. Fred Trump's black-and-white photo sits close to President Trump in the White House oval office as it always had at Trump Tower.

Right alongside his father's ever-observant image sitting on the gifted British wood of the Resolute desk is a black-and-white photo of his mother, Mary. It is a testament to American greatness that Mary, the youngest of ten children, who arrived in America alone at age eighteen after traveling steerage class, now casts her photographic glance at the President of the United States.

Trump attributes his showmanship to his mother. "She always had a flair for the dramatic and the grand. She was a very traditional housewife, but she also had a sense of the world beyond her. I still remember my mother, who is Scottish by birth, sitting in front of the television set to watch Queen Elizabeth's coronation and not budging for an entire day" (Trump and Schwartz, 1987). Several of Trump's books are dedicated "To My Parents, Mary and Fred." Beneath one such inscription is their wedding photograph (Trump and McIver, October 2004). In Trump Tower, directly below his triplex penthouse, he built a special apartment for his parents (although they rarely stayed there, preferring their home across the river in Queens).

Like his "America first" ethos, a psychology of "family first" guides President Trump's response to life's challenges. The murky, ethical conundrum that this view presents to America is amplified further on. But Donald Trump is perfectly clear about it. "There is nothing to compare with family if they happen to be competent, [and] because you can trust family in a way you can never trust anyone else" (Trump and Schwartz, 1987). "My family is very important to me and always has been. I'm happiest when I am with them.... Anyone who visits my office [Trump Tower] will notice that I have many photographs of my family—my parents, my children, and Melania. That's a great positive focus to keep, not that I need reminders, but a glance now and then can keep things in perspective" (Trump and McIver, 2008).

Although the obvious similarities between Kane and Trump help us grasp Trump's fascination with *Citizen Kane* (empire building, wealth, showmanship, Xanadu/Mar-a-Lago, power, and politics), I believe it is the key differences between Trump and Kane that are required to complete his enchantment. Succeeding with love and loss makes everything else worthwhile. Being able to love and bear loss are essential elements in grounding a personality, maintaining stability in the face of life's endless and inevitable challenges and defeats. As the world's most stressful job, the role of president certainly has no shortage of opportunities for challenges and defeat.

Concern about President Trump's public persona being volatile and impulsive must recognize the stabilizing framework of Trump's values of love and respect for loss. They help the dust of frustration settle and bring a grounding perspective. Loss through death or human conflict has been steady in Trump's long life, and I explore the impact of those losses in detail further on. Let us briefly note, however, that President Trump attributes the definitive shift in his mental gears and motivation to be President of the United States to the death of his father, Fred. Additionally, the earlier death of his older brother, Fred Jr., who succumbed to virulent alcoholism, steered Donald absolutely clear of alcohol, drugs, and cigarettes for his entire life.

These very human attitudes concerning love and loss are the bedrock of President Trump's character and must not be lost when captured by his formidable Kane-like persona. And on that note, the notion of "capture" brings us to Reverend Norman Vincent Peale and President Trump's enigmatic rhetoric: Trumpspeak.

CHAPTER

2

TRUMPSPEAK

The story goes that a farmer was selling his excellent mule for ten dollars, but the purchase included a two-by-four wooden plank for an additional ten dollars. The puzzled buyer asked, "What's the two-by-four for?" "Oh," the farmer replied, "that's to get his attention!"

At the age of seventy-two, President Donald J. Trump has the instincts of a millennial. Tweets, America's 280-character equivalent of Japanese Haiku, come naturally and plentifully to him. Attention grabbing hyperbole or outlandish nicknames ("Pocahontas", "Little Rocket Man", "Low-Energy Jeb") ensures our notice. Whether you agree with him or not, you've heard and remembered those names—and may have even quoted them yourself. Gaining access to your thoughts is Trump's first step in persuading you to consider his points. In a crowded stadium, packed with followers, it assures their rapt attention and focus. And as Scott Adams (creator of the popular cartoon Dilbert) points out, attention is an essential element in initiating hypnosis (Adams and Rubin, 2017).

The question arises whether Trump's emphatic hyperbolic style is consciously calculated, intentional, and manipulative. For the most part, I don't believe it is. It's part of his nature, his temperament, and an adult outgrowth of similar traits in childhood.

As Trump said of himself in 1987:

> *Even in elementary school, I was a very assertive, aggressive kid. In the second grade I actually gave a teacher a black eye—I punched my music teacher because I didn't think he knew anything about music and I almost got expelled. I'm not proud of that, but it's clear evidence that even early on I had a tendency to stand up and make my opinions known in a very forceful way. The difference now is that I like to use my brain instead of my fists. I was always something of a leader in my neighborhood. Much the way it is today, people either liked me a lot, or they didn't like me at all. In my own crowd I was very well liked, and I tended to be the kid that others followed. As an adolescent I was mostly interested in creating mischief, because for some reason I liked to stir things up, and I liked to test people, I'd throw water balloons, shoot spitballs,*

> *and make a ruckus in the schoolyard and at birthday parties. It wasn't malicious so much as it was aggressive (Trump and Schwartz, 1987).*

Trump discussed his upbringing similarly on the campaign trail: "Growing up in Queens I was a pretty tough kid. I wanted to be the toughest kid in the neighborhood and had a habit of mouthing off to everybody while backing down to no one. Honestly, I was a bit of a troublemaker" (Trump, 2016).

Although these memories of Trump might sound like those of an incorrigible brat, once he was sent away to military school following months of rebelliousness, he overhauled his personality in a remarkable, self-determined, conscious fashion. He became recognized as a model student and was rewarded with distinguished rank militarily, academically, and athletically. Trump's capacity for sharp verbal retort may have been abated but was not lost.

Later in life we'd see Trump's office door always open at Trump Tower, with his orders, questions, insults, exasperations, and requests shouted out by Trump. Hundreds of daily telephone calls interspersed the constant movement of people in and out of his office. Much of this spontaneous, intense one-on-one human communication, an ingrained way of conducting business, has been channeled into tweeting. Tweeting is not new behavior; it is old wine in a new bottle.

A Verbal Cartoonist

Cartoonist Scott Adams has described the dual realities of his readers (Adams and Rubin, 2017). On the one hand they recognize how outlandish qualities are depicted in Dilbert's office life, but on the other hand, it feels like reality. The cartoon evil of a boss who sends employees off in a space shuttle, gleefully stating it is a "win-win" situation—"if it explodes we decrease employee count"—does not prevent a reader from feeling, "this is just like my company!" It feels real. Similarly, when President Trump tweets videos of Muslim attacks in Europe, it does not matter if they are incorrectly dated or mislabeled. The point is made for his followers—jihadists are trouble. Trump has a talent for using hyperbolic metaphor in speech—he is a verbal cartoonist.

Consider two remarks of President Trump in response to the Senate Judiciary Committee's debate over confirming Judge Brett Kavanaugh. "Da Nang Dick," was his caustic outing of Senator Richard Blumenthal (D-CT), whose legal lecture to Judge Kavanaugh on the consequences of lying seemed hypocritical in light of the Senator's election campaign untruths about his service in Vietnam. "Da Nang Dick!" Meanwhile, Senator Dianne Feinstein (D-CA), who belatedly offered the Senate Judiciary Committee Dr. Christine Blasey Ford's confidential letter that mysteriously appeared in the press, was rebranded "Leaking Dianne Feinstein." If President Trump had visual artistic talents, perhaps he would have shined in a website other than Twitter, something like "One Picture is Worth a Thousand Political Words."

Is Trump Aware of His Rhetorical Techniques?

To some extent I believe that President Trump's heated remarks are calculated, and that includes his tweets. Although urged by his White House staff to reduce or cease and desist his tweeting flurries entirely, he has not. This refusal is a conscious decision. Reince Priebus, President Trump's former Chief of Staff recalled that "[he] and other aides including Ivanka Trump, Jared Kushner, and Hope Hicks, his [former] communications director—regularly tried to convince Trump that his random, often incendiary Twitter messages were self-destructive. I told him, 'Some of it's not helpful, it causes distraction. We can get thrown off our message by tweeting things that aren't the issues of the day'.... Everybody tried at different times to cool down the Twitter habit—but no one could do it.... Even the First Lady weighed in when her husband addressed Congress. After the joint session, we all talked to him and Melania said, 'No tweeting,' And he said, 'OK'—for the next few days. We had many discussions involving this issue. We had meetings in the residence. I couldn't stop it" (Baker, February 2018).

Melania Trump continues to volunteer Twitter advice to the president. In a recent interview in Egypt, in front of the Sphinx, Mrs. Trump volunteered the following advice: "I don't always agree with what he tweets, and I tell him that.... I give him my honest opinion and honest advice. Sometimes he listens, sometimes he doesn't. I have my own voice and my opinions and it's very important to me that I express how I feel." Asked if she ever tells the president to put away his phone, Mrs. Trump quickly replied, "Yes!" (Rogers, 2018). During his time in office in 2017, Trump's total tweeting time neared forty hours (*The Boston Globe*, 12/26/17). In April 2018, his lifetime tweeting total was over 37,000 tweets (Draper, 2018). And by 2019, he's surpassed 40,000 tweets.

President Trump's reverence for tweeting is exemplified by Dan Scavino, the White House's "Director of Social Media" (a new position created by Trump). Scavino first met Trump in 1990 when caddying for him, and still holds the two one hundred-dollar bills that Trump tipped. Trump presciently remarked, "You are going to work for me one day." Indeed, Scavino later joined the Trump campaign, often referred to as "the Conductor." Although his role was opaque to outside observers, he remained in the campaign's inside circle, and now occupies a similar, privileged spot in the White House.

Scavino has a special role in President Trump's tweeting, and Scavino's installation indicates the deep importance Trump attaches to tweeting. Scavino is reputed to have a keen grasp on the pulse of Trump's base and the kind of messaging they need to hear (Draper, 2018). With the departure of Hope Hicks, Scavino has replaced her post outside the Oval Office. President Trump often checks his tweets first with Scavino to solicit input about content or phrasing. Scavino occasionally does the actual posting of the tweet to Trump's account. Scavino also maintains President Trump's Facebook account. Trump, with great pride, views himself as a literary lion of the tweeting world. He has boasted, "Somebody said I am the Ernest Hemingway of 140 characters" (Draper, 2018).

White House staff put effort into mastering President Trump's grammatical style, and often present him with three or four suggested tweets on a pressing topic. Trump will then select the one he favors, at times with no suggested editing, and tweets it out. Like the journalistic army of fact checkers scouring Trump's verbal output for factual errors and distortions, there is also an ardent journalistic endeavor to study his tweets and determine what percent of the tweet was actually composed by the president. Based on all his prior tweets dating back years, journalists have learned that tweets featuring photos, videos, and hashtags are less likely composed by the president. Important is the style of grammar, including misspellings and staccato syntax, since these singular Trump features link him to the everyday voter who put him in office and thereby helps maintain his image as a "man of the people." The White House staff, to their delight, have become exceedingly adept at mimicking Trump's style, and it has become more difficult to spot the tweets that are not pure Trump. Trump's confident spontaneous style of tweet creation has been contrasted with that of former presidential candidate Mitt Romney, who famously required twenty-two staff people to review a tweet. The result was a paragon of grammatical purity, but lacked the impact that only spontaneity can bring (Linskey, 2018).

The widespread impact of President Trump's tweeting goes beyond fodder for scrambling journalists; it now influences the stock market. Traders must check President Trump's tweets which have clear impact on the market (Arends, 2018). In June 2018, Trump's early morning telegraphing that the soon-to-be-announced jobs report would be greater than expected caused the stock market to soar. This action instilled significant criticism as a potential "illegal disclosure."

As opposed to the view that Trump's frequent tweeting represents a discharge of anxiety second to an inordinate sense of vulnerability, Trump feels that tweeting announces that he is not a victim: "[With tweeting] I have access to this great megaphone, I can fight back." He can also set the tone with strategic tweets that are intended solely for the consumption of his core supporters (Begley, 2017). Staid Washington, D.C. has had its communication norms upended by Trump's recognition that Twitter has given him power to maneuver public opinion outside of the mainstream media. For Trump, tweeting is like having a personal publishing empire with no filter. Trump has happily boasted, "It's so great that I have Twitter now. I can now knock the crap out of people....I have my own printing press!" (Draper, 2018). Shades of *Citizen Kane*!

Trump's in-your-face style online is a continuation of his 2016 winning campaign—a campaign fought in many non-traditional ways. Trump trusts what he calls his "gut instincts" above his staff's recommendations.

"The...key to the way I promote is bravado. I play to people's fantasies. People may not always think big themselves, but they can still get very excited by those who do. That's why a little hyperbole never hurts. People want to believe that something is the biggest and the greatest and the most spectacular. I call it truthful hyperbole" (Trump and Schwartz, 1987). "So sometimes I make outrageous comments...to make a point. I'm a businessman with a brand to sell. When was the last time you saw a sign hanging outside a pizzeria claiming 'The fourth best pizza in the world?' But now I am using those talents, honed through years of tremendous success, to inspire people" (Trump, 2016).

Scott Adams has underscored Trump's awareness of the psychology that partly powers his rhetorical effectiveness as revealed in a December 6, 2017 speech in Pensacola, Florida, a Trump stronghold (Adams, 2017). While extolling strong economic news, including a booming stock market with rising consumer confidence, Trump flatly stated, "It's all about psychology to an extent, and that's what makes greatness." Trump's vision—processed through rose-colored glasses and thereby promoting a self-perpetuating rose garden—brings us to a keen fashioner of such lenses, Reverend Norman Vincent Peale.

Norman Vincent Peale

Donald Trump has acknowledged only two people in his life as "mentor," his father, Fred Trump, and Norman Vincent Peale (Kranish and Fisher, 2016). Peale (1898–1993) was the Pastor of the Marble Collegiate Church of New York for over fifty years. A venerable ministry, this reformed church traces its origins back to 1623 and the first ordained minister of New Amsterdam (New York's earlier Dutch name). Located on Fifth Avenue in Manhattan, from late childhood into adulthood, near fifty years, Trump attended Sunday services and heard Peale's sermons. Reverend Peale performed the marriage ceremony for Donald and Ivana as well as Donald's two sisters. A friend to many presidents, Peale even officiated at the wedding of President Nixon's daughter. Trump continued to attend Marble Collegiate Church after Peale's death, which was also the site of the funerals of both his parents.

The Reverend Norman Vincent Peale was a mesmerizing speaker who Trump extolls. "Dr. Peale commanded the pulpit like no one else. He was perhaps the greatest speaker I have ever watched" (Trump and Bohner, 1997). "I especially liked his sermons. He would instill a very positive feeling about God that also made me feel positive about myself. I would literally leave that church feeling like I could listen to another three sermons. I learned a lot from Norman Vincent Peale.... I think people are shocked when they find out that I am a Christian, that I am a religious person. They see me with all the surroundings of wealth so they sometimes don't associate that with being religious. That's not accurate. I go to church, I love God, and I love having a relationship with Him. I've said it before—I think the Bible is the most important book ever written" (Trump, 2016).

When Trump Tower was completed, Peale sent Trump a letter reminding him that he had predicted "You were going to be America's greatest builder.... You have already arrived at that status, and believe me, as your friend, I am very proud of you" (Barron, 2017). Peale was folksy, humorous, uplifting, and like Trump, spoke without notes (only at the end of his presidential campaign did Trump give in to a teleprompter). Trump, in his familiar, self-declarative manner, is unequivocal about his relationship with Peale: "He thought I was his greatest student of all time" (Kranish and Fisher, 2016).

Peale authored *The Power of Positive Thinking*, which was on the *New York Times* bestseller list for 186 weeks. A popular radio personality for fifty-four years, Reverend Peale was also a figure of great controversy. One critic summarized his book as "The Bible of American Auto-hypnotism." It is filled with mantras, prayers to be repeated, visualizations, and is a veritable manual of autosuggestion. But, from a contemporary vantage point, many of the techniques are similar to psychiatrically accepted, modern Cognitive Behavioral Therapy (CBT), and also in vogue with many sports coaches (visualizing a successful effort, like a golf swing, football punt, or diving off a high board).

Here are a few of Peale's counsels, whose words one can hear Trump echoing in his own statements:

> *Formulate and stamp indelibly on your mind a mental picture of yourself as succeeding. Hold this picture tenaciously. Never permit it to fade. Your mind will seek to develop the picture. Never think of yourself as failing.... So always picture "success" no matter how badly things seem to be going at the moment.*
>
> *Stand up to an obstacle. Just stand up to it, that's all, and don't give way under it, and it will finally break. You will break it. Something has to break, and it won't be you, it will be the obstacle.*
>
> *Affirm it, visualize it, believe it, and it will actualize itself.*
>
> *Practice the technique of suggestive articulation, that is repeat audibly some peaceful words. Words have profound suggestive power and there is healing in the very saying them.*
>
> *When they asked an obviously happy aged man his secret to happiness he said, "I haven't any great secret. It is as plain as the nose on your face. When I get up in the morning, I have two choices—to be happy or to be unhappy. And what do you think I do? I just choose to be happy, and that is all there is to it (Peale, 1952).*

Much of Reverend Peale's advice rested on faith in God and scripture: "Believe in yourself! Have faith in your abilities...confidence in your powers...[It] leads to self-realization and successful achievement.... Positive thinking, faith in God, faith in other people, faith in yourself.... If thou canst believe...all things are possible to him that believeth (Mark 9:23). If ye have faith... nothing shall be impossible unto you (Matthew 17:20).... Every problem has in it the seeds of its own solution. If you don't have any problems, you don't get any seeds."

This last positive Pealeism is woven into Trump's accounts of his successes in real estate. He thrived in situations of chaos, seeing opportunities abound in the midst of what looked like failed prospects to others. In his first major Manhattan success, Trump revamped the decaying hotel, the "Commodore," transforming it into The Grand Hyatt against his father's advice. Trump's father, Fred, said, "Buying the Commodore at a time when even the Chrysler Building is in receivership is like fighting for a seat on the Titanic" (Kranish and Fisher, 2016). Just like Peale's wisdom would advocate, Trump was undaunted.

It might be difficult for non-New Yorkers to comprehend the extent of the ugly, frightening, neighborhood decay surrounding the crumbling Commodore and adjacent Grand Central Station, as well as much of New York City in the 1970s. In 1971, the city's hotel occupancy rate reached a low of 62.5 percent. New York City was dying, near bankruptcy, and people who could afford to were leaving. Trump was in the vanguard of turning that deterioration around—which I now realize was his first foray into "Making America Great Again." This time the slogan was "Make New York Great Again!"

In December 2012, in the spirit of the power of positive thinking, Trump tweeted:

> *"'Christmas waves a magic wand over this world, and behold, everything is softer and more beautiful'—Norman Vincent Peale."*

Apart from the cheery mood of Christmas, Trump has drawn on Peale's heartfelt optimism in times of dire adversity:

> *In the early '90s I was in a ton of debt. I had gone from the smartest guy in town to a complete zero. One night I went into the conference room where my accountants were still working, and the mood was definitely stressful because everyone was focused on unpleasant things.... I started describing to everyone all of my plans for future projects and developments and how fantastic they were going to be. I went into detail about them, painting a vivid picture of success. My accountants all acknowledged later that they thought I had actually flipped out.... They thought I had cracked, that maybe I was beginning to hallucinate from the pressure.... But from that moment on, our focus changed from looking at our big problem to looking at our terrific future. Things changed for the better. Changing the focus to what we loved doing was the turning point.*

> *After that I actually started negotiating new deals (Trump and Zanker, 2007).*

He later stated that "Believing that a negative situation is temporary and wrong will give you the impetus to do something about it.... Being unhappy and unproductive is simply not part of my game plan" (Trump and McIver, 2008).

A similar scenario played out during the presidential campaign. In former campaign manager Corey Lewandowski's book *Let Trump Be Trump*, one chapter begins "Donald Trump's chances of winning are approaching zero—*Washington Post*, October 24, 2016; Donald Trump Stands a Real Chance of Being the Biggest Loser in Modern Elections—*Huffington Post*, October 27, 2016; Our final map has Clinton winning with 352 electoral votes—*Los Angeles Times*, November 6, 2016" (Lewandowski and Bossie, 2017). In one of the darkest moments of this unrelenting, bleak, statistical black hole of the presidential campaign, *Let Trump Be Trump* describes a seminal, top level strategy meeting at Trump Tower with key people from Donald Trump's campaign. Among the people present were executive chairman Steve Bannon, New Jersey Governor Chris Christie, and Trump's daughter, Ivanka. Republicans across the country had been urging Trump to drop out of the race, and a number of people in the room were thinking along similar lines. The Chairman of the Republican National Committee, Reince Priebus, presented Trump with two stark choices: "With all due respect, sir, you have two choices. One, you lose the biggest electoral landslide in American history and take everybody with you, or, two, you can drop out of the race and let someone else be the nominee." In the stunned silence of the room, Trump leaned forward, looked Priebus in the eye and said, "First of all, I'm going to win. And second, if the Republican Party is going to run away from me, then I will take you all down with me. But I'm not going to lose." And that was that. Flash forward to the early hours on November 7, 2016, when Trump walked out to give his victory speech. "Sorry to keep you waiting," Trump joked as he took the stage just minutes after securing 306 electoral votes in the election upset of the century.

In 2008, Donald Trump published a book with Meredith McIver titled *Never Give Up*. In it he compiled what he labeled his "Top 10 List for Success." The items on his list are so close to Peale's prescriptions that it worth listing them as they are deeply built into Trump's self-psychology. Despite being written over ten years ago, one can see all these elements of Trump's current rhetoric and conduct. Trump's ten rules include:

1. Never give up! Do not settle for remaining in your comfort zone. Remaining complacent is a good way to get nowhere.
2. Be passionate! If you love what you're doing, it will never seem like work.
3. Be focused! Ask yourself: What should I be thinking about right now? Shut out interference. In this age of multitasking, this is a valuable technique to acquire.
4. Keep your momentum! Listen, apply, and move forward. Do not procrastinate.
5. See yourself as victorious! That will focus you in the right direction.

6. Be tenacious! Being stubborn can work wonders.
7. Be lucky! The old saying: 'The harder I work, the luckier I get' is absolutely right on.
8. Believe in yourself! If you don't, no one else will either. Think of yourself as a one-man army.
9. Ask yourself: What am I pretending not to see? There may be some great opportunities right around you, even if things aren't looking so great. Great adversity can turn into a great victory.
10. Look at the solution, not the problem. And never give up! Never, never, never give up.

President Trump doubters often express concern that Donald Trump does not listen to others. To the contrary, his identification with Reverend Peale is seamlessly threaded through his rhetoric and provides an unshakeable, guiding consistency.

The Social Psychology of Trump's Rhetoric

D.W. Winnicott, a brilliant British innovator in the psychological understanding and treatment of children, famously concluded that "there is no such thing as an infant without a mother, to discuss one, you need the other" (Winnicott, 1958). In the same vein, there is no leader without a follower and no follower without a leader. The leader owes his or her power to being a condensed dream-like symbol of the followers' conscious and unconscious aspirations.

Some political observers were baffled by wealthy Trump's appeal to the broad segment of working people—carpenters, plumbers, painters, roofers, bricklayers, electricians, factory workers, and dozens of other nuts-and-bolts tradespeople who shape our economy. How does this Manhattan billionaire know which words, themes, and style will grab their attention?

Insufficient appreciation is given to Trump's early and continued exposure to everyday forms of blue-collar work. From the time he could walk he accompanied his father, Fred, to work. Fred was a self-made man, learning carpentry in night school as a teenager. When Fred's mother, Elizabeth, formed Elizabeth Trump & Son, he was so young that she had to sign the checks. Starting from scratch, Fred built small, add-on garages himself before moving on to building homes. After many years he knew all aspects of the building trade. He encouraged his son, Donald, to do the same, and he did. Summer jobs for Donald involved laboring at the same kind of jobs his father did before him. After college, Donald spent five years working with his dad in the building trade of Brooklyn and Queens, usually seven days a week. With that immersion in the industry he developed close relationships with many different kinds of people, learning about their struggles, their joys, their sorrows, and most importantly, how they spoke. Trump's bluntness, practical and to-the-point, found reinforcement on the job. This communicative style might be heightened or at times toned down, but its basic nature is now irreducible. Before he stepped his business foot into Manhattan, Trump spent twenty-seven years in Brooklyn and Queens.

"It is ironic that the warrior that they [Southerners] have found is a billionaire from New York, but he really speaks their language fluidly," said Henry Barbour, a Republican National

Committee member and party strategist based in Mississippi. "I don't think it's about any specific set of policy positions, but it's about somebody being a warrior for folks" (Haberman, 2018). Similar sentiments were expressed by attendees at an October 2018 rally in Southaven, Michigan, where people lined up for several blocks five hours before President Trump spoke. "He doesn't try to take his words and make them please everybody, and I think that Southern people are noticing that…[Another said] I don't really look at him as a politician…I look at him as just one of us. He doesn't act like he's above you, as a person." The South is definitely Trumpland, where in 2016 he won every state except Virginia. Recent polling shows that Trump has maintained a healthy 60 percent approval rating in Tennessee. *The New York Times* summarized their view of Trump's Southern appeal: "Southern Republicans have forged a deep, personal connection to the man they saw on television for years. Mr. Trump does the four things those voters love, rally attendees said: He wins, regardless of how fungible the definition of winning may be. He takes the fight directly to Democrats, unlike previous Republican presidential candidates who preferred comity over controversy. He does not bow to politically correct culture. And he does not condescend to them" (Haberman, 2018).

In this balance of leader and adherent there is a significant element of fate. The leader miraculously fulfills the desired role of the followers, but, in truth, he or she can do little other than "be" what is desired and fit into that role. A successful leader is one who can comply with that reality with ease. This performative element of Trump (and most other charismatic leaders) reminds me of the great entertainer Al Jolson, who always insisted that the theater's house lights be turned up when he performed so he could see the faces of the audience.

As a child I saw one of those performances and it was electrifying. Trump does not speak into space—he sees people, notices some flicker of their behavior, and comments on it. That allows his followers to feel seen—no small achievement speaking before rallies of thousands.

An unspoken, powerful social psychological caretaking embrace of Trump's followers, North and South, is conveyed with his daily and often several times daily, tweet-touching of their mental shoulders. Who else does such surveillance of one's life? Such mental alerting usually occurs with parents or loved ones who care. These are desirable, hard-to-come-by, affective undertones in a political communication. Without a middleman, a Trump supporter can respond immediately with replies or retweets. This sort of active engagement replaces the relative passivity of reading newspapers or sitting in front of a TV—the voting populace is engaged. The individual feels as if they're having a dialogue with the President of the United States on a daily basis. From this interactive point of view, in generating political engagement, tweeting beats watching the talking heads of TV or reading journalistic pundits.

Affective Rhetoric is Effective Rhetoric

When President Trump saunters onto a stage in a crowded auditorium or stadium and roars, "What a crowd! The biggest ever!" this is not a mere boast of box office appeal. He is saying through affect and body, "All you people are great! You are here! I love that you came in force and you are a force! You are showing your power, your belief, your determination. You are undefeatable!" When he skirts political correctness with a heavy emphasis on "radical Islamic terrorists," or uses the term "illegal immigrants" as opposed to "undocumented immigrants" he is giving open voice to what he judges is a suppressed public voice, a threat to freedom of speech. As well as stifled speech, Trump is zeroing in on stifled feelings, stifled affect. Unleashing such affect also often unleashes the thoughts attached, the sense of relief becomes attached to Trump. Ironically, often the target of psychiatric slander, Trump is a political healer, an appreciated campaign country doctor. He delivers catharsis.

An extraordinary example of concern over suppression of freedom of speech came from what, to me, was an extraordinary place—*The New York Times*. The *Times* has been an unrelenting, searing critic of President Trump. Yet, on October 4, 2018, an op-ed was titled: "For Once I Am Grateful for Trump: In the president, one big bully stands up to others." The author, Bret Stephens, a longtime, passionately anti-Trump journalist, remarked:

> *For the first time since Donald Trump entered the political fray, I find myself grateful that he's in it. I'm reluctant to admit it and astonished to say it, especially since the president mocked Christine Blasey Ford in his ugly and gratuitous way at a rally on Tuesday. Perhaps it's worth unpacking this admission for those who might be equally astonished to read it. I'm grateful because Trump*

> *has not backed down in the face of the slipperiness, hypocrisy and dangerous standard-setting deployed by opponents of Brett Kavanaugh's nomination to the Supreme Court. I'm grateful because ferocious and even crass obstinacy has its uses in life, and never more so than in the face of sly moral bullying. I'm grateful because he's a big fat hammer fending off a razor-sharp dagger (Stephens, 2018).*

In stepwise fashion, Stephens details how our age-old legal standard of "innocent until proven guilty" was insidiously twisted into "guilty until proven innocent through partisan motivated politics," thus enabling one-sided media attacks on the testimony of the accused while simultaneously treating the accusers with "Faberge egg delicacy" (Jackson, 2018). In making point after point, Stephens expresses his stifled affect unleashed by Trump's untrammeled affect. This is an interesting instance of Trump rhetoric as healing, delivering emotional catharsis in this usually hostile journalistic territory. Trump can connect with individuals who don't like him.

A noticeable feature of Trump's performance—and it was a performance, complete with deadpan pauses—was its occurrence despite ardent appeals from his White House staff to keep quiet on the issue. As we've seen during his campaign and throughout his presidency, Trump, like many of his followers, has deep faith in his instincts, enabling him to ignore accepted political practices. After the Senate vote confirmed Brett Kavanaugh as a Supreme Court Justice, Trump felt convinced that his fiery speech in Mississippi was the turning point in that close, tension-filled, political jockeying. In a reversal, the White House staff who previously were fervently opposed to Trump publicly expressing a strong opinion on this contentious issue, agreed that Trump tipped the scales on the issue (Colvin, 2018). "Establishment Republicans initially reacted with horror. But Trump's 36-second off-script jeremiad proved a key turning point toward victory for the polarizing nominee, White House officials and Kavanaugh allies said, turbocharging momentum behind Kavanaugh just as his fate appeared most in doubt.... 'As long as he was willing to go to the mat for him, it fortified people up here, too,' said Sen. John Thune (S.D.), the chamber's third-ranking Republican leader.... [A White House aide commented] that the president ultimately followed his own gut as if he were 'a strategic boogeyman'" (Rucker, Parker, Sullivan and Kim, 2018). A few days after the Kavanaugh victory, President Trump explained his aggressive attack on Dr. Christine Blasey Ford, "I thought I had to even the playing field.... It was a very unfair situation. So, I evened the playing field. Once I did that, it started to sail through" (Sargent, 2018).

President Trump's recurrent freewheeling attacks on those who oppose him are replete with humiliating nicknames that stick like rhetorical glue, distressingly confounding his critics and media commentators (Baker, October 2018). This aggressive behavior is rooted in Trump's childhood temperament, reinforced through most of his life in the successful use of similar tactics in business, and pleasantly philosophically articulated for him by Reverend Peale. He is playing out Peale's exhortations to stand up to any obstacle, be forceful, envision only victory, and give all to the battle. Trump's rhetoric does not equivocate.

Reverend Peale offered Trump an uplifting moral rationale for his father's more drastic, sub-rosa, business prescription: "Be a killer!" Recall that Peale and his father, Fred are the only ones in Trump's life he accords the revered title of "mentor." Trump began attending Marble Collegiate Church on Sundays as a boy and continued attending regularly through adolescence and young adulthood—during those formative years when one's cognitive abilities grow and mature. Listening to Peale's philosophy during this period of open mental development and what use he has made of them brings to mind a psychological discovery of Benjamin Franklin. In *The Autobiography of Benjamin Franklin*, Franklin describes his pleased amazement in adolescence to discover what his mind was suddenly capable of—enabling him to do what he always wanted. "So convenient a thing to be a reasonable creature, since it enables one to find or make a reason for everything one has a mind to do," he wrote. For the rest of us, however, a knowledge of Peale's "power of positive thinking" provides a verbal framework around which to understand important unchanging features of Trump's rhetoric.

Trump has deep intuition that his gut instincts represent the desires of his supporters. Most of the time, Trump simply acts. At such moments, I imagine Trump in the vein of famed Yankees catcher Yogi Berra when he was asked, "What do you think of when you are at bat?" Yogi replied, "When I'm at bat, I don't think." Perhaps it's no coincidence that Berra was one of Trump's two childhood sports heroes (the other being the African-American catcher Roy Campanella who played for the Brooklyn Dodgers).

Benjamin Franklin, as we have noted, grasped the significance of emotional antennae underpinning human belief. Psychologically, Trump's spontaneous reliance on his instincts causes his followers to feel that his indomitable maverick behavior, consistently repeated, marks him as independent of any political machine. This helps enhance trust and, more importantly, binds voting loyalty. As one of his former, longtime Trump Organization top executive, Louise Sunshine, emphasized, "He is a very strategic, methodical person. Nothing goes by him. He could be giving a speech in Ohio, and he will know what's going on in the right, what's going on in the left, what's going on beyond, and what's going on behind. He has 360-degree sensory engagement" (Laughland, 2016). His tone, his stance, his facial expressions, and his movements grip the audience—the visible experience of his affects.

President Trump's followers previously feel unheard politically, and through his emotional use of words they feel heard. Feelings are first; facts are secondary. This approach has created an industry of fact checkers (who never seem to fact check those on their own side). Although sometimes correct in their fact-checking, these fact checkers are missing the key point of Trump's strategy—eliciting the emotions he wants from his audience. For example, although migrant conditions vary along our southwestern border, and some may actually be unacceptable, when Trump insists things are fine given the lack of Congressional cooperation, his supporters feel he is keeping his campaign promises to control borders. Their feelings are attached to campaign promises regardless of varying facts.

Trump's emotional caricatures, distorted as they may be, are shortcuts for rhetorical routes to the hearts of his listeners. This is also part of why Trump's flouting of "political correctness" is so acceptable to them. People feel shut down, shut out, and unable to participate in political dialogue.

Recent studies of formally Democratic Midwestern counties where Trump showed dramatic turnaround strength in the 2016 election reported "a deep craving for respect among supporters of the president and an enduring resentment toward coastal elites that buoys his popularity." From Kenosha, Wisconsin, one Trump voter explained, "Our culture in Hollywood or in the media gives off the distinct air of disregard to people who live in the middle of the country, as if we have no value or do not contribute to the betterment of society.... It's frustrating. It really wants to make you stand up and yell, 'We count,' except of course we don't. At least not in their eyes." From Erie, Pennsylvania, another voter said that if you "live in a small or medium-sized town, and you would think we were dragging the country down.... We aren't a country just made up of large metropolitan areas." From Minnesota: "I despise Barack Obama. I think primarily because I don't think he thinks very much of people like me. That's just the long and short of it." A summation of these studies concluded, "Trump appealed to the 'forgotten man,' a term his campaign often used, with a message that was infused less with ideology than grievance" (Hohnmann, 2018). I would add, and perhaps more importantly, the message was infused with empathy for the sadness, the aloneness, and the longing of "the forgotten."

And to be sure, this underdog quality is not one-sided. Donald Trump spent many years running his independent businesses with the feeling he was a loner. During his first several years in Manhattan he was constantly met with a disdainful discounting of his ideas and abilities on many early projects. It took several years of a dogged pursuit to purchase the lease rights of the staid Fifth Avenue department store Bonwit Teller in order to build Trump Tower, and Trump recalls being openly laughed at by the owners in this quest (Geist, 1984). Other projects like the West Side Highway blighted railyard conversion into a thoughtful development of riverside buildings, paths, and parks, took twenty years of often humiliating and frustrating negotiations. Both Trump and his audience know work, hardship, and frustration. In that sense, leader and follower are one.

A Good Slogan Concentrates Affect

"Make America Great Again" is aspirational—Peale-like in its appeal—and emotion leads concept. A nostalgic longing for a pastime that is possible once again, but only if we "make" it. Similar to his intuition concerning the underlying sadness in *Citizen Kane*, Trump hones in on what makes affective sense on a national scale. He addresses a nation in mourning for what it has lost, or even worse, allowed itself to lose. Nationalism supersedes diversity—America First. Implicit in this proposition is an unspoken promise of caring. It is as if he saying, "Forget European Allies and foreign treaties. In fact, forget the rest of the world beyond our borders—you come first among my concerns!"

"Great Again" is hope. It is simple and yet every affective word can be expanded into volumes of thought. It draws on the past to create a great future. It depends on the past and invokes it. It brings to mind the words of the distinguished American historian Arthur M. Schlesinger Jr., who worried that America, being born of so many immigrants bordered on being a land of "historyless" people threatening national "disorientation." President Trump addresses that threat with "Make America Great Again," the essence of his rhetoric.

CHAPTER

3

THE PERSONA AND THE PERSON

Carl Gustav Jung

It may surprise people to discover that Donald Trump has read the works of Carl Gustav Jung (1875–1961), the Swiss psychologist and psychiatrist. Jung's analytical psychology has "fascinated" and guided Trump, who says that, "in my business as well as in my personal life…[Jung] keeps my mind open to my unconscious." Trump was introduced to Jung by a friend who had suffered several personal crises, but Trump was impressed that despite suffering personal turmoil, he appeared calm with "grace under fire." Trump inquired as to how he did it. The friend explained that reading Jung had provided an understanding of life that gave him psychological equilibrium and "kept him centered." Trump began reading Jung with great satisfaction. "If someone had told me in business school that studying psychology would be important for financial success, I would not have believed it." He highly recommends Jung's end-of-life autobiography *Dreams, Memories and Reflections* (Jung, 1961). Trump counsels, "[This book] will fine tune your intuition and instincts.... You will gain a technique for seeing into—versus reading into—the people around you.... Jung will give you insights into yourself and the ways in which you and other people operate" (Trump and McIver, March 2004).

The Importance of Persona to Donald J. Trump

The persona is a central Jungian concept. Persona is derived from Latin, where it referred to the mask worn by actors in ancient stage performances. The mask is distinct from the actor who wears it, even if there may be shared characteristics. For Donald Trump, "persona" captures a fundamental component of his personality. Trump explains:

> *Each of us has a persona. We need it for survival. It's the face we put on for public use, and it can be intentional or unconscious. For example, a salesman who has lost his entire family in an accident is, naturally, devastated. But to work effectively with his customers, he must appear cheerful and confident. That is part of his persona.... The only danger is when people become their personae. That means something has been shut off somewhere along the line, and these people*

> *will end up hiding behind the false personality that works professionally.... This hit home...I am aware of my public side as well as my private side, and, while I'm not one for hiding much, I know there are several dimensions in which I operate.... The people I work with day in and day out know I'm not entirely a glam guy. They see how hard I work. One person said I am very much like a Mormon (Trump and McIver, March 2004).*

President Trump's Persona Requires Down Time

President Trump's need for solitude is absent from his public persona. Prior to being in the White House he had arisen at 5 AM and spent three hours reading several newspapers (*The New York Times, The New York Post, The Wall Street Journal,* and others) while simultaneously watching TV news. In the 1990s, those who worked closely with Trump describe him as a "homebody." His attorney, Jay Goldberg, said that the public image of flashy women and liaisons were all carefully staged moments for press photographers.

In *The Art of the Comeback* (1997) Trump explained that "The press had me linked to dozens of women. But, as a friend so aptly stated, I couldn't have built my empire if I was having that kind of action. It was incredible, being intimately associated with women I had never heard of. Women themselves—some very famous—were linking themselves to me.... Their agents were calling. It was a circus! It was sick." Trump names women whom he had met under the slightest of social circumstances who "informed" the press that they were Trump's latest romantic interest. On a Géraldo Rivera broadcast, Trump confronted one who broke down sobbing, admitting "it was a scam."

Of Trump's nocturnal habits, Goldberg said, "Give him a Hershey bar and let him watch television...I only remember him finishing the day [by] going home, not necessarily with a woman, but with a bag of candy." Trump himself has said that at the end of the day he loved walking over to his favorite Korean supermarket for "potato chips and pretzels, [which at times] will be my dinner." Evenings, he often read (favored biographies and numerous magazines), or, watched TV sports or news alone.

Trump's marriage to Melania did not alter his habits. After dinner he still pursued solitary activities, although at times they enjoyed sports TV together. The book *Fire and Fury* (Wolf, 2018) worryingly described Donald and Melania having separate bedrooms in the White House, with Donald retiring to his bedroom around 6:30 PM. Mental eyebrows were raised at this arrangement, but in their social circles it is quite common (Wang, 2017). In Palm Beach, and particularly in Manhattan, due to the high cost of living and consequent expense of apartments, separate bedrooms are a status symbol. President Trump and First Lady Melania Trump's evening routine in the White House is remarkably similar to their life in Trump Tower.

Reading and the Private Self

For President Trump, both ends of the day are bookended by solitude, downtime from the varied, usually frenzied, activities of his persona. Or as he knowingly puts it, in the plural, his "personae." Although President Trump's reported activities in White House evening hours have not included reading literature, it was a regular feature of his evenings prior to becoming president. For example, in a book jam-packed with people and endless daytime activity, *How to Get Rich*, he emphasized:

> *I need a certain amount of quiet time...in order to stay balanced. It's time I use to read and reflect, and I always feel renewed and refreshed by this. It also gives me material to feed my extroverted nature. For me the early morning hours are best for this reflection.... [But also, in the evenings] once I'm home, I read books—usually biographies. Now and then I like to read about philosophers—particularly Socrates, who emphasizes that you should follow the convictions of your conscience.... I tend to agree. It may not make you too popular, but it's essential for lucid thought.... And avoid being part of the herd mentality.... I like movies and television as much as anyone else, but reading is a form of replenishment for me. The potato chips and pretzels help, too (Trump and McIver, March 2004).*

Prior to Trump's campaign for the presidency and his entry into the White House, Trump often received reading recommendations from his oldest sister (age eighty-one), retired federal judge Maryann Barry. He has always been in frequent contact with his oldest sister. One literary recommendation of Judge

Barry's was Aldous Huxley, whose surmounting of physical struggles captivated Trump. "He was such a learner that when he was faced with near-total blindness as a young man [several years as a teenager], he learned braille and continued his studies anyway. His description of this predicament had not a trace of self-pity. In fact, he mentioned that it had offered some benefits: He could now read in bed at night and his hands would never get cold because he could read with his hands under the covers. Learning begets learning" (Trump and McIver, March 2004). Although throughout my long life I considered myself an avid reader and have read several Aldous Huxley books and articles, I never knew about his blindness until I read Trump.

There is a special irony in Trump's interest in Huxley. Counter-Trump interests in dystopian novels have mushroomed during Trump's presidency, and Aldous Huxley's *Brave New World* has climbed back up the bestseller lists. Despite not even appearing in Amazon's top one hundred selling books, in 2017 it vaulted to the top 10 (Wheeler, 2017).

On September 11, 2005, Trump wrote a letter to the editor in *The New York Times* that was later accorded the annual "Best Letter to the New York Times Book Review" by *New York Magazine*. Donald Trump listed some of his reading. "I've read John Updike, I've read Orhan Pamuk, I've read Philip Roth." Pamuk must have been a recommendation of his sister's. Pamuk is a Turkish Nobel Prize winner in literature that I have enjoyed and a compelling storyteller, but his name is hardly one that is on everyone's literary lips. Elsewhere Trump noted that Erich Maria Remarque's *All Quiet on the Western Front* is one of his favorites, and he also gave accolades to two books by Doris

Kearns Goodwin, *Team of Rivals* and the Pulitzer Prize-winning *No Ordinary Time* (Ittalie, 2018). Pre-presidency, books may not have been a leading feature of Donald Trump's life, but they were certainly not foreign to his experience, and he took pride in his familiarity with good reads.

Whatever President Trump's reading habits prior to his campaign and presidency may have been, I have no indication that such reading continued through his presidential campaign until today. The exigencies of the presidency appear to have catapulted him into a fulltime, business modus operandi similar to that of the Trump Organization. In contrast to Trump's nocturnal literary pursuits, at the Trump Organization he did virtually no reading of contracts and agreements, entrusting that assiduousness to loyal, trusted, longtime employees. After their deft to-the-point summaries and recommendations he would either sign a document or send his loyal troops as well as himself back into negotiating battle. In part, I believe President Trump and the former Director of the Central Intelligence Agency Mike Pompeo worked so well together because the unread daily briefings were exactly that—brief.

Reports of White House life in January 2018 describe an increase in President Trump's need and time for solitude (Swan, 2018). This time is categorized as "executive time" by the White House administration. "Trump's days in the Oval Office are relatively short—from around 11 AM to 6 PM, then he's back to the residence. During that time [in the Oval Office] he usually has a meeting or two, but spends a good deal of time making phone calls and watching cable news in the dining room adjoining the Oval Office. Then he's back to the residence for more phone calls and more TV.... Aides say Trump is always doing something—he's a whirl of activity and some aides wish he would sleep more—but his time in the residence is unstructured and undisciplined. He's calling people, watching TV, tweeting, and generally taking the same loose, improvisational approach to being president that he took to running the Trump Organization for so many years." Commenting on this schedule, former White House Press Secretary Sarah Huckabee Sanders has written: "The time in the morning is a mix of residence time and Oval Office time but he always has calls with staff, Hill members, cabinet members, and foreign leaders during this time. The President is one of the hardest workers I've ever seen and puts in long hours and long days nearly every day of the week all year long" (Swan, 2018). Evenings, nights, and mornings provide long stretches of time at Trump's disposal since he claims a lifelong limited need for sleep, perhaps four to five hours. Corey Lewandowski during the long, grueling presidential campaign, described seeing Trump take a nap on an airplane only a handful of times, and that was usually only about thirty minutes (Lewandowski and Bossie, 2017). In the pressure cooker of Washington, Trump has carved out clear expanses of time to safeguard his private self. He has a clear understanding, a workman-like respect for what he personally requires for mental equilibrium. For all his persona's spontaneity, in a disciplined fashion, there is a rigorously held private-self schedule.

The President: A New Brand

Donald Trump has devoted his adult professional life to forging the "TRUMP" brand, a marketable brand that has been the badge of his persona. Over the marketable brand a new emblem is being forged: the presidency. Trump's design of the brand's new feature is partly preconceived, partly intuited, but more importantly, is shaped on the job. Even the *TRUMP* brand was forged on the job. Originally, Trump intended Trump Tower to be called Tiffany Tower, capitalizing on the famed jewelry store right next door to Trump's new skyscraper under construction. A friend of Trump, who works in real estate, suggested to Trump that he not hand off the marketable glow, but instead seize the burgeoning limelight with his own name—Trump Tower. This advertising "Aha!" moment of conversation was the birth of the *TRUMP* brand.

In chapter six, "Substance, Style, And Suitability For Presidential Leadership," I dive into the latest addition to the *TRUMP* brand, the presidency. Elements of the presidential persona's brand are intended to be seen, obvious, open for admiration and acknowledgement—the private self remains protected and hidden.

Protecting the Private Self

Apart from solitude, Donald Trump protects his private self with legal and contractual agreements. For example, in the pre-nuptial agreement with Ivana, in the event of divorce, "Paragraph ten stipulated that in exchange for the money I was to give her, Ivana was not to write any account of our life together or of my business affairs without obtaining my written consent. This included the publication of diaries, memoirs, letters, interviews, and fictional accounts. If Ivana breached this clause in any way, I would no longer be obligated to uphold the financial end of the contract" (Trump and Bohner, 1997). Ivana's recent book *Raising Trump* (2017) avoided intimate marriage details, stuck closely to the rearing of their three children, and received Trump's written consent.

During Trump's 1999 foray into presidential campaigning for the 2000 election, his divorced wife, Marla Maples, threatened to reveal what Trump "is really like" if he chose to run for president in the general election in an interview with *The Daily Telegraph*. Trump immediately withheld alimony of $1.5 million, claiming she violated the confidentiality of their divorce agreement. The conclusion of a thorny bramble of legal and court actions saw Trump pay the alimony, but most definitely the legal hell burned Marla as she did not violate the confidentiality agreement. Non-disclosure agreements (NDAs) are also a standard requirement of employee contracts in the Trump Organization.

As president, Trump has introduced NDAs to his White House administration staff. It is legally questionable whether such agreements would hold up to challenges in court since they impinge on government employees' freedom in discussing non-classified materials, but White House aides have signed the agreement. The terms, quite similar to those employed in The Trump Organization, are "breathtakingly broad" and encompass statements related to "Trump, Pence, any Trump or Pence

Family member, any Trump or Pence company, or any Trump or Pence Family Member Company" (Dawsey and Parker, 2018).

The Washington Post reporters' book *Trump Revealed* (2016) was granted an interview with Trump only after agreeing to no contact with his three siblings. Considering the enormous press coverage of Donald Trump, his wives and children, it is remarkable how little one reads of his brother, Robert, and sisters, Maryanne and Elizabeth. Interestingly, in *The Washington Post* interviews, Trump was described as in control and "would not be pushed." His persona was on exhibition. "He boasted about a great deal, but he mostly kept quiet about what was going on deep inside." The persona briefly subsided when Trump was asked about his favorite film, *Citizen Kane*. The interviewer felt a momentary glimpse into Trump's less seen, inner self. *Citizen Kane* as a choice for his favorite film was no idle gesture and is tied to the emotional values of his personal self, particularly in the tension between the power of love and the power of wealth.

Earlier I outlined the powerful and enduring impact the Reverend Peale had on Trump through his formative years and adult life. Interestingly, Peale echoed a basic split in his own personality, as profound as Trump's split between his persona and private self. The current senior minister of Marble Collegiate Church, Dr. Michael B. Brown, states there were two Norman Peales: "Peale the motivator and Peale the pastor.... A lot of the public thinks Peale the pastor was saying the same stuff as Peale the motivator.... In the motivational speaking world, he would say 'You can if you think you can.' In the pulpit he would quote Philippians 4 and say 'I can do all things through Christ who strengthens me'" (Barron, 2017). Many powerful people in politics and business attended the services of Reverend Peale. After his 1960 presidential campaign defeat by Senator John F. Kennedy, former Vice President Richard M. Nixon worshipped at Marble Collegiate Church.

Archetypes: The Hero-Mentor and Philosopher-King

The Jungian understanding of life entails "self-actualization." A person lives propelled by aim and purpose as well as pushed by the past and heredity. The present is determined not only by the past, but by the future ("Make America Great Again"). Optimally, one continuously strives for a harmonious blending of unconscious and conscious being. Donald Trump emphasizes, "The ego is the center of our consciousness and serves to give us a sense of purpose.... The ego works to keep our conscious and unconscious aspects in balance. Too much either way can be detrimental.... Strive for wholeness" (Trump and McIver, October 2004). We have bountiful evidence of Trump's conscious—just read his daily tweets. But what is in Trump's unconscious mind?

Archetypes

I was intrigued by a brief comment made by Steve Bannon when he was part of Trump's administrative cohort. Bannon commented to Cory Lewandowski (Trump's campaign manager) that Trump explained his shorthand nicknames as "archetypes" (Lewandowski and Bossie, 2017). Examples include "Lyin' Ted," "Little Marco," "Low-Energy Jeb," "Sleepin' Joe," "Little Rocket Man," and "Crooked Hillary," among many, many others. As president we have heard "Leaking Dianne Feinstein," and eventually even ensnaring Bannon himself as "Sloppy Steve." Politics plays a capricious role in shaping Trump's choices. During President Trump's 2018 mid-term election campaigning, "Lyin' Ted" was refurbished for Texas Republicans as "Beautiful Ted" and "Texas Ted." Since President Trump in 2017 still references "archetypes," it is worthwhile speculating what influence they have on him.

Jung described two vast seas of the unconscious. One is the personal unconscious, a repository of past personal experience. The other is the collective unconscious, which contains forces common to all people. This storehouse of human history and experience contains the archetypes. The "archetypes" are amalgams of forces, complexes, seeking expression—actualization. Examples of major archetypes are sage, creator, rebel, hero, and the ruler. One of the major archetypes may dominate personality.

Throughout all of Donald Trump's writings runs a theme of builder as "hero." His real estate projects restore decayed entities (the Commodore and surrounding neighborhood), generate life (acres of Manhattan's Westside Penn Central Railroad Yards laying fallow), awaken potential (Trump Tower), bring vision to blindness (40 Wall Street reinvented), rescue from bureaucracy (Central Park Wollman Skating Rink), and restored a "beat-up, overgrown Rembrandt" (Mar-a-Largo). Most, if not all, of his projects involved Herculean challenges—economic, political, architectural, and cultural. The odds were against Trump, who faced numerous situations where knowledgeable people predicted failure. And some failures did occur, such as his Atlantic City casino bankruptcies. Many of his real estate colleagues were not "heroes." They did not surmount. And many did not survive—Trump did. Some of these friends and colleagues' business misfortunes are detailed in Trump's *The Art of the Comeback*.

Most of Trump's books are framed as mentoring books, including *The Art of the Deal*, *How to Get Rich*, *Think Big*, and *Never Give Up*. Even *The Apprentice* is guidance on how to be the best. A marital mirroring is reflected in First Lady Melania Trump's motto for children: "be best." The psychological force behind the drive to "be the best" is the archetype of the "wise old man."

According to Jung, if one is progressing in self-actualization, the hero—wise old man can meld into the archetype of "philosopher-king." And in this progression, I am sure you can see Trump's mental travels along the road to the presidency. Intuitively, Trump feels he is providing the nation a chance to actualize dormant archetypes. The depth of his belief that he is a political and cultural savior instills great resolve, confidence, and a feeling of virtue in the face of any obstacle.

Consistency is a hallmark of Trump's personality, regardless of what he reveals or hides. It leads in a particular direction, one in which he sees himself as a person who acts, changes, shares, and betters his world. Trump's long-standing interest in Jung gives us a peek into his unconscious. And, the conscious persona is not solely a plastic put-on mask; its best talents grow out of the whole nature of the person, it has roots in the unconscious. The ego balances it all.

The other consistency worthy of note is Jung's view of the human condition, which offers paths to self-actualization. In its murky mythic preoccupations it has an unyielding optimism reminiscent of Reverend Peale.

The Person and Persona in Love

With the women he loved, Donald Trump's relationships have remarkably long lives—as opposed to the relatively anonymous years of fleetingly dating models, actresses, sportswomen, and high society figures.

As Trump himself said, "Prior to my marriage [to Melania], I would go out with a woman that was very beautiful, but if there was no chemistry, no matter what I did, it just wasn't going to work…[One needs]….somebody you can get along with, that you'd be friends with, and that you have great chemistry with" (Trump and Zanker, 2007).

"Great chemistry" created three marriages. With Ivana, the marriage lasted fifteen years, counting a courtship of about six months and then from marriage (1977) until divorce (1992). Marla Maples and Donald Trump reportedly first slept together in 1987 (Hurt, 1993). Six years later they married (1993) and then divorced (1999), a relationship lasting twelve years. With Melania, a steady relationship for near seven years prior to marriage (2005) has lasted twenty-two years and continuing. Fifteen years, twelve years, and twenty-two years (thus far)—Trump's three loves have been sustained, serious efforts.

With Ivana and Marla, the end stages of marriage entailed harsh conflict (personal and legal), and the evaporation of the passion they once shared. By October 1989 it had been sixteen months since Donald and Ivana had sex (Hurt, 1993). Trump disclosed that the divorces were a "hell" that no business turmoil matched. His comments reveal an honesty about divorce and an acknowledgement, once again, that the vicissitudes of love "trump" those of business. The poignancy of lingering love, as revealed in the last line of his following comments, reflects his capacity to face the painful realities of life.

As Trump explains the emotional turmoil of divorce, "You are in love with somebody, and then realize you are in a war. The battle is so intense, far more intense than it gets in a business transaction. There is nothing more vicious than a man or a woman going through a divorce. It is pure hell, like nothing I have ever seen.... As a businessman...[I have experienced] terrible litigation. Deals go bad, partnerships break up, and all hell breaks loose.... It's nothing compared to the fight between a man and a woman, who used to be in love and sometimes still are" (Trump and Zanker, 2007). That statement is a powerful expression of psychological strength, and Trump's ending comment "and sometimes still are" reflects his capacity to feel loss of love while still valuing it.

Despite these purgatorial divorce processes, in several books and interviews Trump has repeatedly extolled the intense love that propelled the marriages and fueled them until they fell apart. President Trump says that he remains friends with his ex-wives, and there's little reason to doubt that. Ivana's second marriage was held at Mar-a-Largo. Marla was at the Republican National Convention in July 2016 witnessing their daughter, Tiffany, speak in support of her father. Both former wives had honored seats at the presidential inauguration of January 2017. Ivana boasted that although she was not "first lady," she was "first wife." Indeed, Ivana has a delightful cameo appearance in the 1996 film comedy *First Wives Club*. Offering advice to marriage beleaguered Diane Keaton, Bette Midler, and Goldie Hawn, Ivana opines, "Ladies, you have to be strong and independent. And remember—don't get mad. Get everything!"

Donald described Ivana and Marla as two extremes of his personality. Ivana was the sharp minded, hardheaded businesswoman who served as interior designer for The Grand Hyatt; CEO of Atlantic City Trump Castle and Casino, and President of the Plaza Hotel. Marla, a model, actress, and singer-songwriter, mirrored his flamboyant entertainer side. One can frame these loves in Trump's Jungian view as pieces of his "personae." And, in this latter sense, this unfortunately kept his private self isolated. This imbalance is a key to the failure of those marriages.

Ivana and Marla are intertwined in Trump's psyche. What first delighted Trump about Ivana is what ultimately repelled him—her expertise as a businesswoman.

Trump explained, "My big mistake with Ivana was taking her out of the role of wife and allowing her to run one of my casinos in Atlantic City, then The Plaza Hotel.... I could have hired a manager.... The problem was, work was all she wanted to talk about. When I got home at night, rather than talking about the softer subjects of life, she wanted to tell me how well The Plaza was doing, or what a great day the casino had.... It was just too much. I work from six o'clock in the morning until seven or eight o'clock at night; to come home and hear more was just not tolerable. And Ivana wouldn't stop.... She had to relate everything that happened in detail [not only for that day,] but everything planned for the following days and weeks. I will never again give a wife responsibility within my business.... I soon began to realize that I was married to a businessperson rather than a wife. It wasn't her fault, but I really believe it wasn't my fault either. It was just something that happened" (Trump and Bohner, 1997). In this latter explanation there is not a tone of blame or a shirking of psychological responsibility, but a respect for each other's nature, and an acceptance, painful as it may be, that each other's needs didn't match.

Unhinged in Work and Love

The unraveling of a marriage to a woman he had deeply loved—Ivana—and a home that included three children, unhinged Donald Trump. Looking back in later years he recognized his loss of focus. "I got a little cocky and, probably, a little lazy.... I wasn't focusing on the basics. I traveled to the spring fashion shows in France. What the hell did I have to travel to Paris for when we have better shows in New York? I began to socialize more.... Frankly, I was bored.... I let down my guard.... [I didn't] work as hard" (Trump and Bohner, 1997).

Real estate details that were usually meticulously and obsessively scrutinized by Trump were left to others. In 1989–1990, following the tragic death of three key Atlantic City casino executives in a helicopter accident, he discovered painful, expensive negligence by others that would have never occurred in Trump's earlier business years. One such case was the construction of The Taj Mahal casino, which, to his surprise, was almost a year and half behind schedule and cost overruns were mounting As a result, this added to Trump's increasingly burdensome debt and delayed his ability to generate the cash flows needed to pay it down. He had neglected the construction process, often looking it over only on weekends. Trump's usual constructing style was modeled on his father's: examine every nail and screw. He had momentarily lost that work rigor. Casino executives left unsupervised by Trump had bungled finances for expensive casino rock star concerts with losses running into the millions (Hurt, 1993). It was in this psychologically unbalanced period that financial recklessness led to his ruinous casino bankruptcies. Trump's mind was elsewhere in an adolescent rebellion from his failing marriage.

In this regressive maelstrom he began his affair with Marla Maples. He lodged her in several of his properties, including the St. Moritz in Manhattan, Trump Plaza in Atlantic City, and even Trump Tower where he lived and worked. Obviously seen by many others, his regressed, out-of-control behavior was that of an unhappy rebellious adolescent telegraphing his trouble to everyone. After one notorious newspaper outing of Trump's love life, his father, Fred, paid him a surprise visit at Trump Tower. In Donald's office his behavior was loudly lambasted by his father, who listed all its dangers, and demanded that he stop. Donald listened dutifully, but his dad left exasperated, feeling he had zero impact on Donald.

Not unrelated to the mentally blinding, regressive pressures of marital failure was midlife failure of his body, increasing weight and flabbiness. He underwent liposuction to remove unsightly fat and had scalp surgery in an effort to stave off baldness (part of the source of his distinctive coiffure).

In short, Donald Trump, humiliated by marital failure, resorted to living out a fantasy that a return to the unrestricted life of his youth would cure his pain. Marla Maples was a Georgia backwoods, hometown, knockout beauty, a blonde pageant queen; he could feel young and invincible again. Marla Maples immortalized Trump in a *New York Post* headline as "The Best Sex I Ever Had." As one pundit noted, this was a "libel proof headline."

The affair lasted twice as long as their marriage. Although Marla Maples pressured Trump for marriage, often bringing her wedding dress on their travels, he was resistant. There were many tumultuous breakups and passionate reunions. Their eventual marriage seemed mostly to be in response to Marla's pregnancy. As Trump commented, "I'm not the kind of guy who has babies out of wedlock and doesn't get married and give the baby a name. And for me, I'm not a believer in abortion" (Zadrozny, 2016).

Marriage to Marla began on an ominous note. Trump later recalled that during the wedding ceremony "I was bored when she was walking down the aisle, I kept thinking, 'What the hell am I doing here!'" (Fagan, 2005). At the time of the marriage in 1993, Trump had moved out of his distracted adolescent retreat and had returned to his former empire-building vigor. Plus, surviving his New Jersey casino bankruptcies required deft financial footwork with absolute focus. The marriage Marla had in mind did not fit that picture.

Conflicting Views of Marriage

In the musical comedy *Guys and Dolls*, Adelaide has spent years pursuing her lover with hopes of marrying, and finally bursts into a witty, sprightly song outlining a new strategy: she will marry him as soon as possible—and then later shape him into a more suitable husband. Perhaps that's what Marla had in mind, but for the two of them, it did not work out that way.

Trump said, "Marla wanted more and more of my time.... Our lifestyles became less and less compatible. We wanted different things. Marla was content when it was just her, Tiffany (their daughter), and me." He also faced complaints such as "Why can't you be home at five o'clock like other husbands?" Donald would protest that her lifestyle would not exist without his work, and besides, he loved his work. He felt unappreciated and misunderstood, often arguing, "Why would you want to take something that I enjoy and change it?" In essence, he concluded, "For a man to be successful he needs support at home, just like my father had from my mother, not someone who is always griping and bitching.... [To be successful, a man] must cut the cord" (Trump and Bohner, 1997). And, cut the cord he did; they divorced after three and one-half years of marriage in 1996.

Interestingly, Trump's romantic trajectory with Marla Maples followed the same course Marla had with Jeff Sandlin. With Sandlin a passionate love begun in high school and endured several stormy, off-and-on-again years. Sandlin complained, "She was always trying to change me [to become a model or actor].... We would have horrible fights.... She slapped me, socked me, and threatened to kill herself." Like Trump, Sandlin, would eventually extricate himself from the relationship (Hurt, 1993).

In marriage to both Ivana and Marla, Trump's private self was increasingly compromised. Home was not a sanctuary from the persona. There was no room to recoup from the day's toil, albeit a loved toil. Ivana wanted more of the persona and Marla wanted less. Both were unfortunately blinded to Trump's private needs. To sum it up in Trump's words, "One thing I have learned: There is high maintenance. There is low maintenance. I want no maintenance" (Trump and Bohner, 1997). Melania provided it.

Seeking Balance

With Melania, Donald has returned home. His mother, Mary Trump, never upstaged or belittled her husband. Yet, as Donald's sister, Maryanne Barry points out, Mary was extremely smart, "maybe one of the smartest people I have ever met." Donald Trump's mother was a powerful presence in the background of his life. Melania Trump is similar. Early photos of Mary Trump glow with the attractive longhaired beauty of a Scottish lass. Melania Trump's beauty is more Manhattanish sexual, stylish—no camera could find her unprepared. The book *Trump Revealed* (Kranish, 2017) reveals that "To Trump's confidants, his third wife's temperament seemed to best balance his perpetual histrionics. 'Of all three women, Melania handles Donald the best,' said Louise Sunshine, who for decades served as a close [business] adviser to Trump. 'She's very independent. He's very independent. She doesn't hesitate to tell Donald good from bad, right from wrong.'" A *New York Times* report in August 2018 (Rogers) stated: "The president does not often accede to anyone's influence, but those close to the family say Mrs. Trump is the strongest voice in the president's life. Several people in the president's orbit have relied on Mrs. Trump to try to get back in Mr. Trump's good graces when they have found themselves criticized or on the outs." Thomas J. Barrack Jr., one of the president's oldest and most trusted friends, elaborated: "He listens to her more intently than anyone and respects her advice and counsel not only because she is his wife, but because her loyalty, grace, trust, elegance under fire, intellect, and instincts are time tested and proven.... He's Donald to her."

The New York Times article also emphasized that "Allies describe Mrs. Trump as warm, engaging and witty, traits at odds with the totemic stance she often takes in public. Just like her husband, she often ignores guidance from aides in favor of her own instincts." Similar to her husband, Melania exhibits a distinct split between her private self and her public persona. Melania quietly matches Donald's iconoclastic social behavior. Summarizing their public life in Manhattan, a Vanity Fair article reported that:

> *'The Trumps don't comport themselves by the rules that are important to people, especially people on the Upper East Side,' says Wednesday Martin, author of a memoir called Primates of Park Avenue, which chronicles the ways of Manhattan's rich and privileged. 'They've rejected out of hand the established rites and rituals of philanthropy—which are to have a cause, have an event, buy a table and get your friends to, and then do the same for them.' New York society ladies paint a picture of a woman with an extraordinary*

> *interest in maintaining her beauty and in this she has succeeded wildly. Even among the devoted SoulCycle set, Melania makes everyone feel dowdy by comparison, says a woman in that circle (Peretz, 2017).*

With minimal explanation or apology, but with great personal dignity and assuredness, Melania concluded life in New York for six months before joining President Trump in the White House. Perhaps the clearest understanding of her psychological empathy for her husband was expressed in this book's chapter "Citizen Trump." That she reveals little publicly concerning her relationship with President Trump is worth noting in the context of appreciating their marriage: "We give ourselves and each other space. I allowed him to do [what he wants], to have his passion and dreams come true—and he lets me do the same. I believe [in] not changing anybody. You need to understand [another person] and let them be who they are" (Kranish and Fisher, 2016). And, "It's a lot of responsibility for a woman to be married to a man like my husband.... We have a great relationship. We are both very independent. We know what our roles are and we are happy with them. I think the mistake some people make is they try to change the man they love after they get married. You cannot change a person. You accept the person" (Wood, 2017). President Trump takes pride in his wife's respect and confidence in him, tweeting on November 28, 2017: "Melania, our great and very hard working First Lady, who loves what she is doing, always thought that 'if you run, you will win.' She would tell everyone that 'No doubt, he will win.'"

Recent stories of President Trump's alleged extra-marital affairs must consider this often-repeated marital stance: "You cannot change a person. You accept the person." Given Melania Trump's intelligence and sophistication, and the public nature of Donald's affairs, it is impossible to believe she has never known anything of them. But during her trip to Africa in October 2018, in a sit-down interview, she did comment on the alleged infidelities of her husband: "'It is not [a] concern and focus of mine. I'm a mother and a first lady, and I have much more important things to think about and to do. I know people like to speculate and media like to speculate about our marriage...' Asked if she's been hurt by the allegations, Melania said, 'It's not always pleasant, of course, but I know what is right and what is wrong and what is true or not true'.... Asked by ABC News if they still have a good marriage and if she loves her husband, the first lady replied, 'Yes, we are fine.... It's what media speculate, and it's gossip. It's not always correct stuff'" (Stracqualursi, 2018).

After over twenty-two years of being together, Donald and Melania have established their marital accommodations. There is currently no evidence that President Trump has engaged in extra-marital relationships either during the 2016 campaign or in his tenure at the White House. President Trump has stated that campaigning had "changed" him, and certainly, his Evangelical base has taken him at his word and continues to support him (Borchers, 2018). President Trump requires a balance between his public persona and his private self. Does he have that balance with his marriage to Melania? He has said, "Anyone who has ever met [Melania] will never forget it. She's just as beautiful on the inside as she is on the outside.... She is a very calm and soothing person who has brought a sense of stability to my very turbulent life. I am lucky to be with her!" (Trump, March 2004). And although Trump thought about running for the presidency off-and-on for perhaps three decades, it was only with Melania by his side that he actually did it, and did it successfully. Yet, we know little of the intimate details of Trump's "private self" directly. Most of what we know is deduction from his numerous writings, the media, reports of friends, or from business contacts. Melania also says relatively little of their private life, but she and Donald have been together for over twenty-two years. That says a lot.

CHAPTER

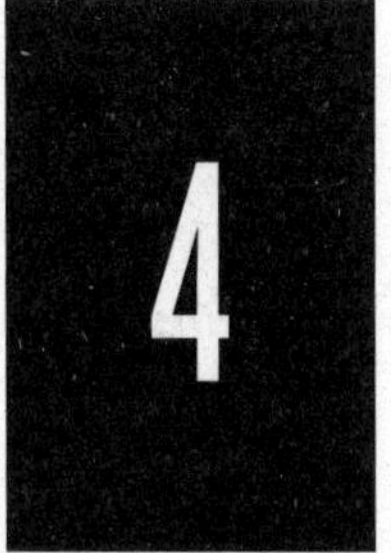

THE LESS VISIBLE TRUMP, PART ONE

A Blurred Beehive

Donald Trump is a complicated man—his brand persona always on display. Trump's multi-layered relationships with family, friends, acquaintances, and businesspeople are less clearly seen. Since Trump's personas' features spring from his nature, what appeals to the masses is recognizable in Trump's less visible world.

People Grow Under Trump's Umbrella

The Trump Organization has many employees who have been with the company twenty to thirty years, and a few who have been with the company since its inception in 1980. In those years many developed into key figures. Norma Foerderer (1929–2013) began with Trump in 1981 as a secretary. By the time of her retirement twenty-six years later she was a vice president. When she started there were seven employees of The Trump Organization. Currently, there are 22,500 worldwide. At retirement, Ms. Foerderer gave her first and only interview (intimates of Donald Trump are protectively closedmouthed):

> *Donald can be totally outrageous, but outrageous in a way that gets him coverage. That persona sells his licensed products and his condominiums…. The private Mr. Trump, on the other hand, is the dearest, most thoughtful, most loyal, most caring man…. That caring side inspires loyalty and is one of his secrets to his success…. [Once he trusts you] He allows you to do purchasing…Human Resources…screening mail…phone calls [eventually, several hundred a week]…PR…research on preliminary projects…. [Even negotiations, which Trump bragged about] Well, I learned from the master. I got him really wonderful deals for commercials. What did I do? I would sit tight and say, 'I want a million.' They'd say, 'Start lower.' My response would be, 'Look you're getting Donald Trump, and there's only one of him, I can't [go] lower…. You're getting a bargain.' I'd just talk and talk and talk, and joke with them. And before you know it, bingo! I'd be just as surprised as anybody else*

that it happened. But I just knew that I had to persevere the way he does (Kessler, 2015).

Foerderer's tactful, frank honesty with Trump was essential to the trust he had in her: "As I came to know him, I realized that Donald is a tremendous man, and I admire him enormously, but if I disagree on something, I would be the first to say to him, 'Donald, I don't think so.'" Foerderer felt that this acceptable forthrightness from those he trusted was fundamental to his success.

Requested for advice to others to succeed, Foerderer said, "I would tell them to dream, and to have a vision and a goal. Think about what you want to do, love it, and if you love it enough, you'll realize your dreams. That's what Donald's done" (Kessler, 2015). The rhetorical arm of Reverend Peale has a long reach.

Matthew Calamari caught Trump's attention at the 1981 United States Tennis Open when, as a security guard, Trump admired his handling of a raucous spectator. He was hired on the spot. He has risen to executive vice president in charge of building operations and runs the entire security organization of the business. At times he has taken charge of major building projects like the transformation of The Delmonico Hotel into Trump Park Avenue.

Vinnie Stellio, starting as Trump's bodyguard, is now a vice president at the company. Trump has said, "Vinnie would often drive executives, architects, and contractors up to Westchester to look at developments I was building. Now they report to him. I am perhaps the largest owner of land in Westchester County, and it's Vinnie who keeps his eye on it all" (Trump and McIver, March 2004).

Meredith McIver, a former ballerina, began as a media assistant in 2001, and eventually co-authored five of Trump's books.

Brooklyn born Allen Weisselberg began with Fred Trump Sr. in 1971 as an accountant fresh out of college, and is now the Trump Organization's chief financial officer. Intimate with all Trump's financial details, the entire family sees Weisselberg as fiercely loyal and steadfastly passionate in his devotion to Trump and the Trump Organization. On January 11, 2017, it was announced that Weisselberg would serve as trustee at the Trump Organization alongside Eric Trump and Donald Trump Jr., while the company's former CEO occupies the Oval Office.

Rhona Graff began as an assistant to Norma Foerderer over twenty-five years ago. Replacing Norma Foerderer upon her retirement was Rhona Graff, who is now Senior Vice President. Formally, she was a popular presence on the *The Apprentice*. Her role has taken on major strategic proportions since Trump has departed for Washington, D.C. She remains in Trump Tower, acting as a powerful, effective gatekeeper for Trump's business. A veritable Manhattan chief of staff, if you will. Across the nation and the world, many who seek access to Trump attempt it through Rhona Graff.

These employees are just a few of the many who have ascended professionally working with Trump. Loyalty and talent (in that order) are valued and rewarded by Trump.

As Trump himself says, "Of course, it takes talent to deal with me and everyone else every day (but especially me)....I don't like it when people underestimate me, and I try not to underestimate anyone else, either. People are multifaceted, and it's important to let them function in a way that will allow them to shine. Most people would rather succeed than fail, but sometimes the leader has to be the catalyst for putting "success" into their personal vocabulary. In other words, try to see beyond a person's title" (Trump, March 2004).

Open Ceiling for Women

Women hold the majority of executive positions in the Trump Organization despite accounting for 43 percent of its workforce in 2015. Their pay was also equal to men (Sellars, 2015). This is an astounding fact for the real estate industry, a brazenly male-dominated realm; especially in the years Donald Trump developed his empire (beginning in 1971). But, in this business appreciation of women, Trump reflects loyalty to his lineage.

It was Trump's German-born, paternal grandmother, Elizabeth Christ Trump (1880–1966), who started her own real estate company when her husband, Friedrich, suddenly died in the great influenza pandemic of 1918 and left her with three children in Queens, New York. Fred Trump was five months shy of his thirteenth birthday at the time. Working as a seamstress and stenographer to make ends meet, within a few years, she formed a real estate entity named Elizabeth Trump & Son (along with her son, Fred). This name was changed only many years later in 1971 to Trump Management after Donald Trump joined the firm after college and it became unclear who the "& Son" now referred to. Elizabeth always remained active in the business, and in her seventies still worked collecting coins from the washing machines and dryers in their buildings in Queens and Brooklyn. Elizabeth's sharp intelligence, talent, business sense, and powerful familial embrace are family lore. Through her grandson, Donald, she has cast a wide influence on women who never knew her.

Similar to Grandmother Elizabeth's harsh challenges, in Germany, Donald Trump's great-grandmother Katharina Trump (the mother of Friedrich) was left with six children and severe debt upon the sudden death of her forty-eight-year-old husband in 1877. In another example where the Trump family overcame economic gender barriers to combat hardships, Katherina mobilized her children and ran a wine business—not exactly the career path expected of a woman in 19th century Germany. And, we shall soon discuss the juristic and banking successes of President Trump's two sisters, retired federal judge, Maryanne Trump Barry, and retired banking executive, Elizabeth Trump Grau. Trump's support for women in business is inherent to his psychology and has powerful roots in his family history.

Barbara Res first caught Trump's admiring attention in the 1970s when she was a construction engineer, on Trump's reconstruction of the moribund Commodore Hotel into the Grand Hyatt Hotel in the decaying Times Square-Grand Central Station neighborhood. For the prior ten years Res had often been the sole woman working with men in construction. At the completion of the Grand Hyatt Hotel, Trump made Res an offer she couldn't refuse. Against all advice and warnings from the real estate world, including his father, Fred, who insisted it could never work, Trump offered Res the role of construction manager in building Trump Tower. Res says, "You know he really did change New York.... [The Grand Hyatt and the Grand Central Station neighborhood] rejuvenated that whole area of the city. It became a destination, that hotel was terrific.... He really had a lot of vision. So, when he told me he was going to do something fantastic on Fifth Avenue, I had every reason to believe it would be so.... So, it wasn't a surprise to me. What was a surprise to me was that he wants to put me in charge. That was a real surprise to me" (Harwell, 2016).

Barbara Res did a magnificent job shepherding Trump's creation of a New York landmark building, and then worked for the Trump Organization for nearly twenty years, becoming vice president in charge of development. Fred Trump never ceased to give Res a hard time during her entire tenure—he telephoned her constantly with quibbling complaints and criticisms. To quiet his father, Donald fudged the sources of her salary so that it was understated to avoid his father's nagging insistence she was unsuitable and not worth the attention his son bestowed upon her. On the other hand, Donald's mother, Mary, greatly approved of Res and was openly supportive, which Res deeply appreciated and acknowledged. Res also noted: "He [Donald] didn't treat women any differently than he treated men. As far as his employees were concerned, he yelled at all of us. The way he treated you had more to do with whether he respected you than it did as to what your gender was" (Harwell, 2016).

Louise Sunshine, an executive vice president at the Trump Organization for fifteen years, stated that she appreciated Trump's "mentoring.... From the standpoint of being a woman, I just thought he was phenomenal.... [Donald] was so supportive and encouraging.... He gave me the ropes, and I could either hang myself or prove myself" (Sellars, 2015). Of Louise Sunshine, Res says, "[Donald] used to have a set of speaker phones on the desk and you would just hit the number and your voice would come over the speaker phone. Louise used to call him on the speakerphone constantly [when we were] having a meeting or whatever and she had this grating voice and it would [blare] 'Donald!' [Donald would plead] 'Louise, I'm in here with people.' 'Well, I need to do this now, you know.' Louise was very tough. She was definitely the strongest woman the guy ever dealt with in business." (Sorry to disappoint Nancy Pelosi, but she has not been the first "tough" woman in President Trump's life).

As documented earlier, Donald gave his first wife, Ivana, extraordinary managerial power on several major projects, including his *Mona Lisa*—The Plaza Hotel, fashionably and romantically located at the corner of Central Park South and Fifth Avenue in full view of Trump Tower. When she was in charge, Ivana took full viewing measure of The Plaza's front door activities from the windows of the Trump penthouse in Trump Tower early every morning. Any out of order activity was fiercely brought into line upon her arrival. Nikki Haskell, a friend of both Donald and Ivana, said, "It was unheard of for a businessman in those circles to give his wife, his new wife, someone who wasn't somebody who had been around for a while, such great responsibilities." Louise Sunshine adds, "[In those days] many rich men didn't allow their wives to come to the office. Many women didn't even know what their husbands did" (Kranish and Fisher, 2017). Ivana was a major force in the design of The Grand Hyatt, then CEO of Trump Castle in Atlantic City (arriving daily for a full work week by helicopter from New York), and finally, president of The Plaza Hotel in New York.

Trump never embarked on a program of fostering women's status in the working world. Diversity wasn't something he actively sought out just for the sake of diversity—it was a natural byproduct resulting from his familial inheritance—and thus became inherent to his business nature.

There's No Place Like Home

On Friday, January 20, 2017, when he was inaugurated as president of the United States of America, Donald Trump had spent almost fifty years in the business world. The mirrored kaleidoscope upon mirrored kaleidoscope of human relationships and contacts is dazzling and incalculable. Trump was a hands-on, super-detailed, "buck-starts-here" and "buck-stops-here" entrepreneur. He signed all checks (profits went down seven percent the only year he didn't, so he began signing them again) and passed judgment on all details, from brass doorknobs to the color of stones on a golf course. Like his father, Fred, Donald personally examined each detail of a building in design and then in construction. He visited sites daily and would climb the stairs of skyscrapers examining railings, doors, knobs—virtually everything he could see. He was constantly exchanging information with accompanying architects, supervisors, and especially the hands-on workmen. The workmen loved him, offered him their opinions, and he always listened seriously. Their opinions mattered—which was a telling detail.

Consider the number and range of relationships encountered in building national and international skyscrapers, hotels, and housing developments with parks and playgrounds; casinos; seventeen golf courses in the United States and abroad; a shuttle airline between Boston and New York; fourteen TV years of *The Apprentice*; merchandising of clothes, beverages, and virtually anything you could put the label "Trump" on; America's major beauty pageants; authoring and co-authoring eighteen books; and making public/charitable/political/ forays as well as endless radio and TV appearances. The extent of such connections is truly innumerable.

Although it was more than thirty years ago, let's not forget the rebuilding of New York City's Wollman Ice Skating Rink in Central Park. Trump voluntarily rescued the rink from New York City's bungling. It had been six years, thirteen million dollars were spent, and yet still there was no restored rink. Trump did the job in four months and 2.4 million dollars—far ahead of schedule and under budget considering the city gave Trump a budget of $3 million and six months. Appreciating Canadian reverence of ice hockey, he consulted Canadian ice-skating rink architects for guidance. Who else would know more about ice than Canadians, after all? Typical of his building style, he could think outside the box and the job was done to New York City's happy acclaim.

This maelstrom of relationships varied from transient to enduring, from disposable to indispensable, from indifferent to loving. Yet when asked about "friends," Trump answered:

> *Well, it's an interesting question. Most of my friendships are business related because those are*

> *the only people I meet.... I mean I think I have a lot of friends, but they're not friends like perhaps other people have friends, where they're together all the time and they go out to dinner all the time.... [Whom would you turn to with a personal problem or doubt about something you had done?]...[That would more likely be] my family.... I have a lot of good relationships. I have good enemies too, which is okay. But I think [I would turn] to my family more than others (Kranish and Fisher, 2016).*

As mentioned earlier, Trump has unequivocally stated, "You can trust family in a way you can never trust anyone else."

The Wall of Family

Given the grounding importance of family in Donald Trump's emotional balance, it is not surprising that his move to the White House entailed installing key family members in his administration. Trump spent his entire life in New York City apart from several semesters as an adolescent in military school. And of that metropolis, only in three boroughs—Queens, Brooklyn, and Manhattan. In this urban gestalt his surrounding family was easily embraced. He brought his philosophy toward family life into business life and ultimately into the White House.

In Trump's childhood, beginning as a toddler, Fred Trump took young Donald along to building sites, and this intimate collaboration never ended. Summers in adolescent years were spent on construction sites with his father. While in college

Donald began a major housing development in Cincinnati with his father which Donald then managed and later sold. Donald described:

> *Fred C. Trump wasn't the kind of dad who took us to the movies or played catch with us in Central Park.... Instead, he'd take me to his "Let's make the rounds," and we'd be on our way. He never yelled at me or had to punish me, but he was always strong, and a little remote, until I joined his business. That's when I really got to know him. I saw how he dealt with contractors and unions, and how he made the most out of every space.... He could be a showman, too. His deals were front-page news in the Brooklyn newspapers. His gift for promotion rubbed off on me.... My father always trusted me. He'd been in business for fifty years, but he'd never let anyone else in the company sign his checks until I came to work. He had absolutely no doubt about my ability. His faith gave me unshakeable confidence.... My father gave me... knowledge...knowledge that became instinctive (Trump and McIver, October 2004).*

Fred Trump, although engrossed in work, was reliably regular—at work at six in the morning, but home every evening for dinner with his family. He and his family also unfailingly attended church every Sunday. Similarly, Trump's first wife, Ivana, says that "Donald didn't know what to do with the kids when they were little. He would love them, he would kiss them and hold them, but then he would give it back to me because he had no idea what to do" (Trump, 2017). The children looked back on their early years with Trump with a sense that they were loved, but a certain sadness that his energies were directed to business. Fred Trump worked seven days a week. On Sundays he'd leave directly from church to check on his latest projects.

Donald John Trump Jr.
1977–

Donald Trump Jr., Donald Trump's oldest son, recalled:

> *It wasn't a "Hey Son, let's go play catch in the backyard" kind of relationship.... It was "Hey, you're back from school, come down to the office." (The upstairs home was only an elevator ride away from the downstairs office.) So, I would sit in his office, play with trucks on the floor in his office, and go trick-or-treating in his office. So, there was a lot of time spent with him, and it was on his terms.... He never hid from us, he never shied away, but it was on his terms. You know, that tends to be the way he does things (Kranish and Fisher, 2016).*

Notice that Donald used the same example as his son, Donald Jr., did to depict a father's relationship with his son—"he never played catch."

At age fifteen Donald Jr. had a tense, bitter, angry, and distant relationship with his father for the year following his father's hotly contested divorce from Ivana. Adding public insult to familial injury, Donald Jr., an adolescent, had to endure the daily, lurid media circus feeding on his family's painful turmoil. At school, this exposure led to many verbal and physical brawls. But, like his father's experience before him with Fred Trump, once Donald Jr. entered the business, a mutual love, admiration, respect, and trust blossomed. Embarking on the presidency, President Trump left the Trump Organization in the hands of Donald Trump Jr. Given the detail oriented, controlling nature of Donald Trump, this handing over of the business reins is a profound and powerful endorsement of his eldest son. This validation, reflecting deep trust and love, is not lost on Donald Jr., who in every interview shines with an unshakeable faith in his father.

Ivana Marie "Ivanka" Trump
1981–

In her recent book *Raising Trump* [2017], President Trump's first wife, Ivana, describes her intense relationship with her own father. "I was a Daddy's girl.... Ivanka and Donald's relationship growing up reminded me of mine with my father." This affectionate memory references a mother's role in fostering a "daddy's girl." Like her two brothers, Ivanka grew up in the Trump Organization, leading her to spend a lot of time with her father. She unabashedly identifies herself as a "daddy's girl," and has worked to create a brand for herself as an entrepreneur in a proud mirroring of her father. She prides herself as being "on a construction site in the AM" and "home for dinner" with her family in the PM. In her two published books there is a theme demonstrating that she's a problem solver who provides solutions (to working women), quite similar to Trump's previously described persona as "hero." "When it comes to business, whatever it is I'm doing, I'm incredibly dedicated to creating solutions for modern women who are living full, multidimensional lives" (Tolantino, 2017). Again, Donald Trump has gifted his children the lesson from Reverend Peale that all problems contain the seeds of their solution.

Eric Frederick Trump
1984–

Similar to his father's childhood, Eric Trump joined his father on work sites early in life, watching, learning, and eventually laboring at various jobs just like his father did with his own father. Eric describes his teenage years as composing of summers spent cutting rebars, hanging chandeliers, and renovating estates in Westchester, New York. Eric says, "He made us work.... And I think that is what a great father does." Like his siblings he has served as an Executive Vice President of the Trump Organization and loves working in the family business. During a key part of his adolescence Eric gratefully accords parental guidance to his older brother, Donald Jr., who he feels offered him substitute fathering since Donald, from Eric's words, "worked twenty-four hours a day." Eric and Donald Jr. remain intensely close. Unlike his siblings and father who all attended the University of Pennsylvania, Eric chose Georgetown University. As a college friend noted, "Eric has Trump genes, but he doesn't have the Trump brand.... I've always admired that he is uniquely his own in that way. Less bombastic, more thoughtful. Less self-aggrandizing, more humble. Less Trump. More Eric" (Zak, 2018). Others have observed the opposite—that Eric shares his father's hyperbolic speech. Despite whatever trauma he experienced during his parents' divorce at just eight years old, it did not follow him into adulthood. In regard to his father, he unabashedly states, "He doesn't have a bad bone in his body" (Zak, 2018). Immersed as deep as one can get in the Trump Organization, and having worked as hard as he could in the presidential campaign from early childhood, Eric Trump has happily joined the Trump family dynamic of loving union through work.

Tiffany Ariana Trump
1993–

Tiffany Trump (Donald's daughter with Marla Maples) has had her early relationship with her father affected by distance because soon after the divorce, Marla has lived three thousand miles away in Los Angeles. Following in the footsteps of her father, Donald Jr. and Ivanka, Tiffany attended the University of Pennsylvania. Tiffany now attends law school at Georgetown University, where Eric graduated having majored in finance and management. Notably, she shows no inclination to follow her mother's Hollywood path as a performer. At the 2016 Republican National Convention, she was a warm, personable speaker in support of her father, and this appearance also established her as part of the first family constellation.

Children as a Priority

Trump has stated that he always took telephone calls from his children at work in Trump Tower. In many transcripts of Trump Tower interviews, one reads of interruptions by children's telephone calls or unannounced walk-ins (because Trump traditionally kept his office door open). Invariably, he stops the interview and attends to his children's calls or visits. Initially, in the White House continued a similar open availability of the president, especially walk-ins. As part of later organizational changes, former Chief of Staff John Kelly halted this disrupting pattern and spontaneous appearances in the Oval Office dropped off radically.

A Good Name is to be Chosen Rather Than Great Riches–Proverbs 22:1

Before adding President Trump's youngest child, Barron, to the family dynamic, it's worth pondering Trump's name choice. During the heyday of Trump's tempestuous and generally affectionate relationship with the New York newspapers, especially *The New York Post*, he often called the papers with gossip about himself, usually disguising his identity over the phone as his own fictitious publicity agent, John Barron. During his affair with Marla Maples, messages to her were often coded "from The Baron." Trump would also occasionally sign them in to hotels as Mr. and Mrs. John Barron. In a never finished film project with a screenwriter titled "The Tower," Trump had only one condition—the main character had to be called John Barron. Donald has said that he always loved the name Barron and wished it were his. The only actual person named Barron that Trump has known and admired is Barron Hilton, the real estate tycoon. However, Trump's use of the name long predated him ever meeting Barron Hilton face to face. It is another intriguing angle of his marriage to Melania, that in this union, he obtained his wish for this name by bestowing it upon his last son. The name represents special feelings and wishes for young Barron on Donald's part, and no doubt will influence this boy.

Barron William Trump
2006–

As of writing, Barron is thirteen years old. Like Trump's other children, Barron has had to adapt to a busy father. His father's busy schedule during his business career would pale in comparison, however, to what it became once he began campaigning for (and became) president. Melania has been a very present mother in his life, keenly overlooking the daily details of Barron's life. Indeed, Barron is fluent in Slovenian, his mother's native language, and converses with his Slovenian grandparents in that tongue.

Alluding to his taste for dressing in suits just like his father, Melania has referred to Barron as "little Donald," and "mini

Donald." Barron also shares his father's enjoyment of golf and building. After trips where certain buildings sparked his imagination, at home, he will sit and sketch drawings from memory. Barron has expressed a desire to be a builder and businessman like his father (Tavani, 2018). With such early in life aspirations modeled on his father's worldly activities, Barron resembles Donald's early childhood modeling of his own father, Fred Trump. Donald and Fred had an intense relationship, a loving bond, based on business not matched by his other siblings. Coupled with Barron being a lifelong name desire of Donald this early modeling suggests a special intense relationship between the two. All of Barron's older siblings came to merge with Donald Trump at later points of development, particularly as they were young adults and joined the family business. I would speculate that this recapturing of his loving bond with his own father through his relationship with Barron is an additional stabilizing factor for the president in the foreign soil of Washington.

Although always appropriately dressed and well mannered, Barron is given sufficient, good-natured leeway to yawn during his father's speeches (which happened during Trump's acceptance speech as Republican candidate and at the inaugural speech). As much as possible, both Donald and Melania have tried to give Barron the privacy his young life deserves. So, we'll have to wait to see the developing nature of this father-son relationship.

Action Speaks Louder Than Words

The point here is a simple one—Donald Trump has given his children what he has received and valued from his own father.

As Donald has said, "My father loved his work.... He was a very content person. He was happy and content. He had a wonderful wife. He had a good family.... So, he would not say [to me] 'work, work, work,... But I would see that he enjoyed what he did. And I learned that way not so much by his words but by his actions'" (Fisher and Kranish, April 2016). "I love relating to [my kids] just the way my father related to me—through a passion for work well done" (Trump and McIver, October 2004).

Trump is intuitively articulating a basic psychological mechanism through which identifications are built into one's character, that action speaks louder than words. Early in life as well as heeding the words of those most important to us, we consciously and unconsciously mirror their behavior, their actions. And enduring mirrored traits—identifications—become an indelible part of who we are.

Beginning with Grandmother Elizabeth one hundred years ago, the Trump family is now in their fourth generation of greasing the family wheels of love, loyalty, and attachment. Most businesses in the United States are family businesses, but only 30 percent survive into the second generation. Barely 3 percent of family businesses survive to the fourth generation. President Trump has a fine cobweb of business ties to all his children and vice versa. Economics becomes so vitally important in the Trump family dynamics not just because it is lucrative, but also because for the Trumps, it is a successful way of loving. One doesn't often conceive of love stoking business success, but it seems to be the case for the Trumps.

And Mother....

Mary Anne MacLeod Trump
1912–2000

Donald Trump's experiences with his mother are more of a mystery than those with his father. Mary Trump was described by her eldest child, Maryanne, as "one of the smartest people I've ever known," but was "tight-lipped." In deference to Fred Trump, she kept herself in the background. With her children she was seen as the disciplinarian, often threatening spanking (imagine managing three boys and two girls) but never following through, and got her five children to toe the mark within the house.

Three women were Mary Trump's beneficiaries—Norma Foerderer, Rhona Graff, and Hope Hicks. They each exhibited Mary's winning combination of sharp intellect, physical attractiveness, disciplined organization, desire to stay out of the limelight, and affectionate devotion to Donald Trump. And as we shall see, each, like a loving mother, threw a daily organizational shawl over Donald Trump.

Mary Trump grew up in grinding Scottish poverty, the youngest of ten children. At age eighteen, alone on a freighter, she immigrated to a bleak, economically depressed America in 1930 to serve as a domestic and nanny. Her first language was Gaelic, and she learned English to attend school in Scotland. Despite an incomplete education, she made an impression on Barbara Res as "A classy kind of person...she had the most polish [compared to Fred Sr. and Donald]." Louise Sunshine, a former vice president in the Trump Organization, described Mary Trump as "a very strong woman...quiet, not aggressive...

loving and embracing" (Kranish and Fisher, 2016). Mary Anne McLeod Trump became an American citizen in 1942. Mary's grandson, Eric, said of her, "My grandmother was an amazing woman who was strong, smart, charismatic and incredibly loving. She had an amazing smile and an incredible sense of humor" (Kruse, 2017). Discussing his mother, Donald Trump is invariably brief and concise, but always enthusiastically portrays her as "loving," "very warm," "a loving homemaker," "loyal," "beautiful," and "fair minded." He also described her as having "a sense of the world beyond her," as being "a great judge of character" and "one of the most honest and charitable people I have ever known," and "supportive" in every crisis he endured. He attributes his showmanship to her "sense of pageantry and glamour" (Fisher and Kranish, June 2016). That President Trump views her as the source of "my religious values" is no doubt reflected in her succinct life advice to him: "Trust in God and be true to yourself" (Trump, 2015).

In all the accounts given by childhood friends of the Trump children, I am struck by three recurring features: (1) friends were always well fed, often staying over for dinner, which entailed the entire Trump family sitting down together; (2) they always felt welcome; and (3) there was always entertainment. Quietly presiding over this relaxed, tension-free atmosphere, in the background was Mary Trump overseeing it all. Outside the home she was active in volunteer hospital work, charities, and the family, often riding in a rose-colored Rolls Royce through the boroughs of Brooklyn and Queens to collect coins from the Trump Management apartments' washing machines and dryers.

During his childhood Presbyterian education, Mary Trump gave Donald a bible that he would always treasure and would later carry with him through the presidential campaign. When sworn in as president he carried two bibles—Abraham Lincoln's inauguration bible and his mother's.

Only in America

Mary Trump never lost her loyal passion for the English homeland, often visiting her home village in later years. Her daughter, Maryanne, counted twenty-four trips with her mother back to her native Scottish village. Imagine the heart swell of feeling flooding Donald J. Trump as he, her son, lived out his mother's deepest dreams when he and Melania came to Windsor Castle for tea with Queen Elizabeth on July 13, 2018. Trump confided to Piers Morgan of the *Daily Mail,* "Well, first of all, I was thinking about my mother. My mother passed away a while ago, and she was a tremendous fan of the queen. She thought she was a woman of elegance, and my mother felt she was a great woman.... I remember, even as a little guy, if there was any kind of ceremony to do with the queen, my mother would be watching the television—she wanted to see it.... I was walking up [to Queen Elizabeth]...and I was saying to Melania, 'Can you imagine my mother seeing this scene?' Windsor Castle.... She'd be very proud.... [Trump told Queen Elizabeth] 'You know, my mother was your big fan. She was born in Stornoway in the Hebrides. And that's very serious Scotland, as you know'" (Edwards, 2018). As we all know, fulfilling one's mother's dreams is serious love.

Father

Frederick Christ Trump Sr.

1905–1999

Fred Trump's relationship with his son is so closely tied to virtually Donald's entire life that we have been exploring their bond since the first chapter. This influence itself is reflective of the power and ubiquitous presence of their love. As has been outlined by the mix of love and work among other family members, Donald and his father loved each other through work. At Trump Management, their mutual passion and dedication to business was seamless and their relationship thrived in that fortunate setting. Outside of business, one special part of their relationship was Fred's discipline. Although Mary has been lauded as the disciplinarian in the family, a similar orderliness came from Fred—and not just in business. Remember, it was Fred who staunched Donald's burgeoning adolescent uprising by harnessing that impulsiveness in a military school. School authorities noted that Fred visited his son more than most fathers, and during those visits often went off campus for dinner together. A few years later, when Donald received sports offers from colleges, it was his father who diverted this path and urged him to attend a nearby Jesuit-run school, Fordham University, in the Bronx. Donald complied, two years later transferring to University of Pennsylvania for business studies.

The presidential apple did not fall far from the family marketing tree. Fred Trump was not shy of public expression, certainly in promotion of his real estate. A popular Brooklyn newspaper *The Brooklyn Daily Eagle* was to Fred's real estate marketing efforts what Twitter is to Donald. Fred was inventive in marketing. On one occasion in 1939 he sailed a Trump branded yacht along Brooklyn Coney Island beaches advertising his properties. Since the vessel was also blasting *God Bless America* and *The Star-Spangled Banner*, the beachgoers stood to salute! They were almost equally unified in their frenzied rush to the shoreline to gather swordfish shaped balloons carrying coupons redeemable for up to $250 toward the purchase of a Trump property (Horowitz, 2016). Fred also spoke highly about his son's abilities. "I gave Donald free rein, he has great vision, and everything he touches seems to turn to gold.... Donald is the smartest person I know" (Klemesrud, 1976).

A Postcard

At the end of a day of work at Trump Tower, once he was alone, Donald Trump often pulled out a box he kept inside of his desk. In that box is a treasure trove of meditative contemplation where Trump keeps special letters, articles, photos, and one postcard. Whenever he picks up that postcard sent to him long ago by his parents, he always feels how much he misses them, he feels sadness and love. It is no wonder Trump grasped the profound meaning of "Rosebud."

Other Bricks in the Family Wall

Fred Trump Jr.
1938–1981

One extraordinary brick in the family wall is "Freddy"—Fred Trump, Jr.—Donald Trump's older brother who died of severe alcoholism in 1981 at age forty-three. Freddy, who was eight years older than Donald, had embraced him as a loved, younger brother, taking him on camping trips, teaching him fishing. It was Freddy's picture that hung on Donald's wall in military school, handsome and dashing beside an airplane. Freddy was the only person that Donald regularly called "honey." "He was the most handsome guy you've ever seen, and he had the best personality of anybody you've ever seen," Donald would say of his older brother (Fisher and Kranish, April 2016). Fred Jr. clashed with Fred Sr. and became an airlines pilot instead of a builder. Donald shared his father's disparagement of Freddy turning his back on the family business, once saying to Freddy in a comment he later came to regret, "What's the difference between what you do and driving a bus?" Perhaps Donald Trump's later foray into owning an airline was a belated apology and show of alliance with his beloved brother.

Donald stated that, "Freddy was an amazing influence [on me] because I don't drink and I don't smoke.... He was a big force.... [Repeatedly] telling me this stuff [alcohol and cigarettes] is garbage.... And so, I've never had a glass of alcohol, and I've never had a cigarette.... It obviously had a great effect on me because I have never had a longing [for it].... And who the hell knows," Donald has speculated that due to his personality, it's very likely that he too could've eventually succumbed to alcoholism without Freddy's advice (Fisher and Kranish, April 2016).

Trump has always been open about his lasting love for Freddy and sadness over his death. Toward the end of Freddy's life his parents sheltered him, but even that could not halt his downward spiral toward a death from alcoholism. Not long before Freddy's death, Fred Sr. described to Donald his frightened dismay looking in Freddy's bedroom closet, discovering that it contained a chaotic heap of empty whiskey bottles. When President Trump gave a major speech on our national opioid crisis in October 2017 he shared the profound impact Freddy's addiction had on his own life and the family who loved him, including the president.

Maryanne Trump Barry
1937–

As mentioned earlier, Judge Maryanne Trump Barry is President Trump's oldest sister. An attorney, she recently retired from her successful position as Senior United States Circuit Judge of the United States Court of Appeals for the Third Circuit, which has jurisdiction over Delaware, New Jersey, and Pennsylvania. Judge Barry is a favorite of Donald Trump. Throughout their entire lives they have been in constant contact—by phone, mail, or frequent family gatherings. Judge Barry is a woman of high intelligence and energy who entered law school after thirteen years of raising her son as a homemaker. During her first job as a lawyer she was one of two women in a sixty-two lawyer firm. After a prominent career as a trial lawyer, she was nominated by President Ronald Reagan and won confirmation in 1983 to become a federal judge in the U.S. Court of Appeals for the Third District. Donald Trump was open about making telephone calls to influential people in support of his sister's application for a judgeship, and when pressed to explain his coercion, candidly stating, "I'm no different from any other brother who loves his sister."

Judge Barry has had a distinguished judicial career, but is extremely private about her personal life. Donald Trump has commented: "I have a sister who just doesn't want to talk to reporters. Can you believe it?" He said that after recounting a time he had called his sister and suggested that she speak with an inquiring reporter and she refused. "Maybe they mixed us at birth. Maybe one of us got mixed up a little bit. Who knows" (Horowitz, 2015). By stark contrast, in the courtroom Judge Barry was known as "blunt," possessor of a "razor-sharp wit," "direct," and, like her brother, disregarded political correctness. Despite their lifelong close relationship, Judge Barry's courtroom decisions reflected strikingly different political views from her brother Donald: she was pro-choice and very pro-immigrant. Donald felt that she was outstandingly supportive and loyal to him during his financial crisis, saying that "She was there in spades" (Rose, 1992). Donald Trump also turned to his sister, Maryanne, for advice after his controversial remarks concerning Megyn Kelly during the presidential debates. Trump has always had an open ear for his oldest sister's words, and by all accounts, they appear to be rendered quite judiciously.

Robert Trump
1948–

Donald Trump had a long history of competition in his relationship with his brother, Robert. Being two years younger than Donald, Robert was quietly accepting of his subordinate position, rebelling only much later in life when he was middle aged. A favored family anecdote from his childhood comes from when he was building with blocks with a young Donald. Donald had "borrowed" some blocks from Robert, and was so serious about his building that he glued his blocks together. Robert never saw his "borrowed" blocks again. Nonetheless, in later life when Robert tired of his life away from family while working on Wall Street, he joined the Trump Organization. Donald Trump was thrilled and felt Robert "had finally come home." Robert moved into an important executive position, and admired his brother's business acumen. Unlike many of Donald's critics, Robert dismissed the idea that Donald was only rich because of his father. In writing his obituary for Fred in the *New York Times* in 1999 obituary, Robert wrote, "but what [Fred Trump Sr.] lent to Donald was mostly knowledge; Donald really did it on his own, along with whatever boost he got from being Fred Trump's son, of course" (Rozhan, 1999). The boost was having Fred as a father—not his wealth.

During Atlantic City's casino financial crisis and after Donald Trump's three key executives died in a helicopter crash in 1989, Donald turned to Robert to take charge. Neither of them grew up in the casino world, but there they were, in a struggling industry in a dying city, in charge. Robert, for the first time in his life, fought with Donald—repeatedly. Over time, Robert withdrew himself from the Trump Organization. The exact details are unclear since Robert, quite unlike his brother, Donald, is very private and far from the purview of the media (except for a high-profile society divorce a number of years ago). Robert moved from New York City, upstate, to Millbrook, New York in the Hudson Valley, where he says he is "gainfully retired." Despite this, he still manages Trump Management, the large real estate business created by Fred Trump through Elizabeth Trump & Son. During Donald Trump's 2016 campaign, Robert Trump reemerged publicly in Millbrook to campaign for his brother in a locality that was hardly conservative. During the Trump presidency Robert has become more public and forthcoming about his brother, always speaking in praiseworthy tones—even when the issue is a bit bizarre. For example, during the imbroglio between former Vice President Biden and President Trump as to who could best whom in a fight, Robert extolled the president's superior athletic ability, effectively telling any bookies out there that Trump is the favorite. In return, Donald unfailingly speaks well of Robert.

Shortly after President Trump's European trip in July 2018, he spotted his brother, Robert, in an assembled crowd and made his way over to warmly embrace Robert and receive a brotherly kiss from him. President Trump added, "Why weren't ya on the stage? I told ya to get up on the stage" (u/narf8h1, 2018). Despite conflicts of the past, their affection runs deep.

Elizabeth Trump Grau
1942–

Elizabeth Trump Grau, four years older than her brother, Donald, is the most private and unknown sibling. Now retired, she had a successful banking career with Chase Manhattan Bank in New York. Unlike Robert, she never entered a Trump family business either with Donald, Fred Sr., or Robert. Of course, she has always shared in the profits of Trump Management, the real estate empire left by Fred Trump and managed by Robert Trump. She married film producer James Grau in 1989, and Donald was an usher at that wedding. Elizabeth raised James Grau's son from a prior marriage, but there were no further children. In print, Donald speaks of her lovingly, but not revealingly. In a Charlie Rose interview in 1992, he did single her out for loyalty to him when he was facing financial crisis. "She was tremendous," he told Rose. Although historical facts are relatively scarce about Elizabeth, her visual presence is not. She is a regular at family gatherings, and was particularly close to Mary Trump right up to her death in 2000. She's a mystery, but as far as Donald is concerned, she's still a sturdy brick in the family wall.

For many years, down the road from their brother Donald's Mar-a-Lago, resided the two sisters, Maryanne and Elizabeth. The two had lovely beachfront homes close to one another. Also living nearby was Maryanne's son from her first marriage, Dr. David Desmond, a clinical neuropsychologist. This close geographic senior Trump family grouping was altered only very recently with the sale of Marryanne's home (Burke, 2018).

Life is With People

Just as Donald Trump has made his mark on the world of real estate with concrete, steel, and glass, his emotional construction is built of people. As Trump noted of *Citizen Kane,* wealth does not guarantee satisfaction in life. Happiness requires love, and love in its myriad variations requires people.

CHAPTER

5

THE LESS VISIBLE TRUMP, PART TWO

The Boss's Mirror

Mary Trump and Fred Trump Sr. were married for sixty-three years. The two also had enduring relationships with others outside the family. Fred's immediate assistant for fifty-nine years was Ms. Amy Luerssen. He had lunch with her daily at Gargiulo's restaurant on his business home turf in Coney Island, Brooklyn (around the corner from Nathan's Famous hot dogs and the boardwalk). In Ms. Luerssen's later years Fred often drove her to the airport, and when her apartment house elevator broke down, he had workers carry her up twelve flights of stairs (Horowitz, 2017). Amy Luerssen continued working with Trump Management after Fred's death in 1999. Amazingly, she continued working into her nineties for the firm. Donald Trump knew her since his early childhood. Like his father, Donald attended to details of her extra-work life like an adored, elderly aunt. *The New York Times* 2006 death notice stated, "The Trump family mourns the passing of our beloved Amy, a trusted and loyal friend and employee for over sixty-five years. A great lady we will never forget, she will surely be missed by all of us whose lives she touched. The Trump Family" (Death Notice, 2006).

Donald developed a similar relationship with Norma Infante Foerderer, his administrative assistant and gatekeeper in Trump Tower, but fate cut them off at twenty-seven years due to Foerderer's sad loss of vision. Norma sat directly outside of Donald's office, a gracious but discerning greeter and filter. If you wanted Donald Trump you first encountered Norma Foerderer, no matter who you were, the governor, business tycoon, sports or media celebrity, down to a walk-in job applicant. One can tell a great deal about a boss by the person who represents them to the world. In a sense, it is what you want people to feel about yourself, a first impression, a setting of the stage, a framing of the portrait.

From the Norma S. (née Infante) Foerderer 2013 Memorial Book at The Frank Campbell Funeral Chapel in Manhattan (Guest Book, 2013), consider these comments:

> *"I'll never forget the name Norma Foerderer. I never saw her face but I received a sincere and*

> *complimentary reply, on gold lettered Trump stationery, to a proposal.... It was such a caring and warm letter...even if they were unable to underwrite the proposed project...an empowering letter, obviously straight from the heart."*
>
> *"Norma, you taught me that it is okay to be terrific at your job and still be nice. Thank you for being such a wonderful mentor to all of us who were lucky enough to be in your magic. We will miss your style and your charm."*
>
> *"Indestructible, wise, classy, always right with her advice and [never one to ever say] 'I told you so.'"*
>
> *"Norma was my personal Audrey Hepburn—a beautiful blend of savvy, kindness, grace and style. Such a LIGHT, that darling woman!"*

In *How to Get Rich,* Trump said an essential for success was to "Ask God for a great assistant. No joke. A great one can make your life a whole lot easier—or in my case, almost manageable. If you want to know what a great guy I am, just ask her. But not on a Friday. Handling me, the office, and several hundred calls a week isn't easy. She's as tough and smart as she is gracious. She's also indefatigable, which helps a lot if you work for me" (Trump and McIver, March 2004).

Similar to a daily White House briefing, the first thing each morning, Foerderer set clippings before Trump that she had culled from newspapers and magazines concerning him or the business. A Manhattan variation on the two-headed god, Janus, Foerderer was a lens through which Trump saw the world for

Trump and alternately faced the world as his surrogate, a surrogate loved, respected, and trusted. It is not sheer coincidence that a person with such admirable traits was Trump's representative. Through Trump's long, valued, loving trust, and reliance on Foerderer, we glimpse pieces of Trump's personality not easily seen. As his emissary she contrasted all his brash personae with tact, open kindness, respect for others' boundaries, willingness to help/mentor/guide, selflessness, and a host of other positive features suggested in the loving notices posted in her memorial book.

Rhona Graff, hired by Foerderer in 1987, spent decades working for her and now fills her stylish administrative shoes and is built of similar material. Rhona Graff, interestingly, has a Master of Arts degree in psychology, knowledge, no doubt, quite suited to the psychological challenges of the Trump Organization.

Trump likens his long relationship to Rhona Graff, now in its fourth decade, to that of his father's with Amy Luerssen. Like Foerderer, Rhona Graff was stationed outside of Trump's open door audibly available for his shouted questions, requests, and exhortations. Also like Foerderer, Graff is tactfully close-mouthed and avoids interviews or public comments. Fulfilling Trump's primary requisite of loyalty, Graff has said unequivocally, "I would never leave him."

With Trump in The White House, Graff has additionally become a judicious conduit for the new flood of inquiries more properly referred to the White House, always relayed by her to White House aides and not the president. Innumerable pieces of Trump's private life are still entrusted to the judgment of Graff. For example, issues concerning the three-story Trump penthouse high above the old Trump Tower office is under her watch as well as judgment as to which telephone callers are further linked to President Trump in Washington. Graff remains the central administrator for the Trump Organization, which is now headed by its trustees—Donald Trump Jr., Eric Trump, and CFO Allen Weiselberg.

Keeping these two trusted women in mind, essential to Trump's sense of security and organization, we can see how the president's recently departed communications director, Hope Hicks, fit into the picture. Similar to Foerderer and Graff, Hicks remained in the background while always up-to-date on the plans and needs of her boss. Like them, she labored long and intensively for Trump, and adored him. And, similar to Foerderer and Graff, people praised Hicks, professionally and personally (Nunzi, 2018). All three women garnered well-deserved trust, respect, and love from Trump.

We are all like the people we love. Those three women shine light on the shadows in Trump's personality—a form of psychological slight-of-hand common to us all. Look at Foerderer, Graff, and Hicks, and you see a side of Trump hidden by his persona.

Respect Nurtures Relationships

Trump is often depicted as an irreverent maverick with little respect for the norms and standards of others, a person so keyed into himself that he cannot understand or empathize with others. However, to those he deems worthy, even those who counter him, Trump's respect and instinctually canny adaptation is central. The first, and no doubt, the most powerful instance of this adaptation, which fosters learning from others, occurred with his father, Fred.

In *The Art of the Deal,* Trump outlined the bitter conflict between his brother, Freddy, and his father. "My older brother, Freddy, the first son, had perhaps the hardest time in our family." Freddy disliked Fred Sr.'s business intensely. "He never had a feel for real estate. He wasn't the kind of guy who could stand up to a killer contractor or negotiate with a rough supplier.... There were [angry] confrontations between [father and son continually].... Freddy usually came out on the short end.... Freddy [to Fred Sr.'s dismay] went off to pursue what he loved most—flying airplanes." Unfortunately, Freddy's professional aviation life eventually unwound along with his marriage. Broken, in his forties, he returned to his parents' home. Despite being received with love and care, he died there wracked by alcoholism.

Trump says he was fortunate in that he was attracted to the construction business from early life and "had a relationship [with his father] that was almost businesslike." He found that he garnered deep respect from his father when he stood his ground on business matters and demonstrated his knowledge. Trump has pondered of his father, "I sometimes wonder if we'd have gotten along so well if I hadn't been as business-oriented as I am."

The bond between Donald and his father was usually transacted through business lines for as long as Fred lived. Donald's eulogy at his father's funeral in 1999 began with him telling the attendees that "My father taught me everything I know. And he would understand what I'm about to say. I'm developing a great building on Riverside Boulevard called Trump Place. It's a wonderful project" (Horowitz, 2016). Embedded, like a special jewel, in this earnest expression of love by a son for his father is a Trump essential—loyalty.

A similar pattern of relational respect for those deemed worthy emerged in military school. At the beginning of his new educational home, Trump continued his irreverent behavior for which military school was the supposed remedy. Then he met Theodore Dobias, a former Marine Corps drill sergeant. With Dobias he learned "about channeling my aggression into achievement."

In a 2016 interview Dobias was described as "nearly ninety [years old]," but with a memory that was "diamond-drill sharp." In the interview he offered remembrances of the adolescent Trump, "I had a lot of one-on-ones with the fourteen-year-old Trump...some of which got physical [fighting]." Dobias did whatever it took to seize the attention of Trump's eighth grade self, and by the ninth grade Dobias seemed to finally have an impact. Trump won the Proficient Cadet award twice, Neatness and Order medal twice, and was accorded Honor Cadet four times. He also played softball and bowling, and received varsity letters for baseball, football, and soccer. Based on his outstanding performances, in 2005, New York State Military Academy inducted him into its Sports Hall of Fame. This interview also quoted a classmate's recollections: "He was just the best, a good athlete, a great athlete...He could have probably played pro ball as a pitcher. I think he threw 80 miles an hour. I was the catcher. He made my hand black and blue every day...Could he play football? Could he play soccer? He could do anything he wanted. He was physically and mentally gifted."

Dobias said that Trump excelled in baseball in particular. Trump was made cadet captain and was a star first baseman for Dobias's varsity squad. Dobias remarked, "He was a good-hit and good-field; we had scouts from the Phillies to watch him, but he wanted to go to college and make real money" (Peebles and Macadaeg, 2016). In another interview, Dobias added: "He did well enough that he was scouted by the Boston Red Sox, a coach at West Point, [and the Phillies].... He became cadet captain because he got along with everybody. He and I got on pretty good. He never got into any trouble" (Bates, 2015).

Trump has shared respectful and admiring reminiscences of coach Dobias: "He was very tough and very rough, the kind of guy who could slam into a goalpost wearing a football helmet and break the post rather than his head. He didn't take any back talk from anyone.... I used my head to get around the guy. I figured out what it would take to get Dobias on my side. In a way, I finessed him. It helped that I was a good athlete, since he was the baseball coach.... What I did, basically, was to convey that I respected his authority, but that he didn't intimidate me. It was a delicate balance. Like so many strong guys, Dobias had a tendency to go for the jugular if he smelled weakness. On the other hand, if he sensed strength but you didn't try to undermine him, he treated you like a man. From the time I figured that out—and it was more an instinct than a conscious thought—we got along great" (Trump and Schwartz, 1987).

Bring in The Marines

Dobias was not the last marine to bring order into Donald Trump's life. Chaos reigned in the White House until the appointment of four-star Marine general, John Kelly, as chief of staff. Not long after Election Day, Trump had asked Senator Tom Cotton, an Iraqi war veteran, who Cotton thought the best general of his generation. Cotton named the conservative, battle-hardened, General John Kelly (Flegenheimer, 2018). After interviews, Trump nominated Kelly as Director of Homeland Security. Before the congressional hearing for that appointment, a colleague suggested to Kelly that he should strategically pin the American flag to his jacket lapel. "I am an American flag!" retorted Kelly. That comment captures a full-bodied, Trump-like self-assuredness that must have been part of President Trump's initial attraction to him.

Prior to Kelly's imposition of order, the Oval Office was run in a manner akin to Trump's office in Trump Tower. A visitor once was stunned at the Trump Organization's disarray and likened the business scene in Trump Tower to "an ongoing family quarrel." Donald's office door was always open; some people strolled in and out, communications were old school, just shouted down the halls.

The White House was initially run like Trump Tower, with the door to the Oval Office left open. Unannounced, people of all rank and station wandered in and out. Rep. T. King (R-NY) described one bill signing in the Oval Office scheduled for a few minutes that ran more than an hour, "It was like Grand Central Station, every White House character was in and out of there" (Rucker, 2018). Flegenheimer relates, "During one Oval Office meeting Trump had with New York Times reporters in April 2017, no fewer than twenty people came and went" (Flegenheimer, 2018).

One of John Kelly's initial actions was to close the Oval Office door. Literally; no one gained entrance without his approval. Prior to Kelly's arrival, endless uncoordinated, unauthorized streams of information were fed to President Trump. Kelly stopped the disordered communiqués. It was rumored that President Trump, in an effort to get around Kelly, starting having meetings in the evening in his bedroom. Kelly's stern authority, however, was such that people feared going around him and kept him informed. The secret meetings stopped (Gill, 2017). Over time, a comparatively relative semblance of order was imposed on the White House administration—but always remained an uphill battle for the vigilant Kelly. This controlling imposition of order also applied to close members of President Trump's family, much to their dismay. Trump's grudging, but respectful, adjustment to Kelly's military orderliness is pointedly reminiscent of Dobias' martial regimen in military school. Unlike military school where graduation released Trump from Dobias's influence, Trump was unable to continue adjusting to Kelly, whose tether broke in disagreement over Trump's contested planned military withdrawal from Syria. Interestingly, the red line for John Kelly was a military decision he could not countenance. Perhaps if he were still a general he would have had a moral, ethical, and military rationale to just "follow orders."

Past is Prologue

President Trump's ability and capacity to compromise with respected, powerful personalities appears in a clear developmental line from his father to Theodore Dobias, and for a surprisingly long time, with John Kelly.

This history of compromise is important to bear in mind when considering President Trump's often seemingly intransient political positions. It reveals a capacity for recognition and respect for competence that engenders productive change in outlook and behavior. These diplomatic leanings are obfuscated by Trump's political persona. His political persona makes grandiose demands with an uncompromising demeanor. Yet in reality, Trump is scouring to make a good deal. Author Mike Cernovich deftly conceptualizes this extreme position—Trump establishes "an anchoring bias," and from there negotiates his way down (Cernovich and Rubin, 2016). This negotiation style was seen during trade negotiations with Mexico and Canada, which were overly beneficial for the U.S. Something similar is in process with Kim Jong un. Initially President Trump talked in terms of "nuclear buttons," which then amazingly faded into pronouncements of "love" for the North Korean ruler. Visions of a dark nuclear war were replaced by promises of peace and prosperity. Recall the futuristic travelogue video President Trump had prepared for their first joint meeting, depicting the paradise that the hermit kingdom could become.

In Trump's account of managing his relationship with Dobias he referred to instinct—"it was more of an instinct than a conscious thought." This intuitive sense of decision making permeates much of Trump's behavior and speech. Trump's reliance on instinct has frightened and concerned the White House administration and much of our nation. In the business world, Trump's instinct was informed by decades of experience. In contrast, Trump obviously doesn't have decades of experience as president. Does President Trump's intuitive style in Washington D.C. reflect a level of experience appropriate for the challenges of the presidency? The predictive dilemma of this dichotomy between a lifetime of personal business experience and President Trump's spontaneous lurches on political and diplomatic terra incognita will be clarified only by history.

Friendship in the D.C. Maelstrom

Dismay is regularly expressed at the frequent dismissal and record turnover of White House staff. People worry that President Trump will be increasingly isolated by "yes men"—those who only mirror and amplify his views. The Trump less visible to the public, the more private Trump, has continued to maintain communication with friends outside the White House. Just like at Trump Tower, his frequent use of the telephone remains a daily aide, a reliable route, to keeping in touch, and its use is often confined to the privacy of his White House bedroom. Emblematic of this resource, and perhaps its most enduring example, is President Trump's thirty-two-year friendship with American-born of Lebanese parents, self-made billionaire (his father had a small grocery store opposite MGM studios in Culver City, CA), Thomas J. Barrack Jr.

Thomas J. "Tom" Barrack Jr.

1947–

Despite his friendship with Trump, Thomas Barrack has never shied away from disagreeing with him. Barrack opposed many aspects of the Trump platform, including the wall, global-excluding nationalism, immigration bans on Muslims (Barrack, fluent in Arabic, is Christian, and American-born of Lebanese parents), and the blockade of Qatar. Barrack has earned Trump's respect and trust through an amazing array of accomplishments, including success in international finance, a sterling track record for economic and political predictions, successful real estate partnerships, financial wizardry in Hollywood, and raising record funds ($100 million) for Trump's inauguration. Barrack also helped Trump out during his aforementioned past business failures. As friends, they have shared feelings over family deaths, divorces, remarriages, and children of similar ages.

Trump finds Barrack's standing in the real estate community impressive. In *Fortune* magazine in 2005, he said, "[Barrack was] arguably the best real estate investor on the planet today" (Kranish, 2017). Trump has admiringly said of Barrack, "He has the discipline of an animal in the jungle" (Jaffe, 2017). It's an interesting word choice for a metaphor due to the fact that Trump made his fortune in the concrete jungle of New York City.

Add to this package Barrack's assertion that he never asked anything of Trump, and even eschewed offers of government or cabinet posts. While he refused political positions, Barrack still embodies the trait that Trump treasures the most—loyalty.

Barrack introduced candidate Trump on the final night of the 2016 GOP convention, and it was Barrack whom he asked to oversee his presidential inauguration. Many who want President Trump's ear seek out Barrack as a go-between. Senator Roy Blunt (R-MO) said, "I've talked to [Barrack] about things I've thought he would be a good person to talk to the president about.... Tom Barrack has a capacity to disagree that others might not have" (Kranish, 2017). Barrack says that although Trump listens and absorbs, he may ultimately hold to his own opinion. Barrack quotes Trump differing with the quip, "I love you, but if I listened to you, I'd still be on *The Apprentice*" (Kranish, 2017).

Roy Marcus Cohn
1927–1986

Another undeniably powerful influence in President Trump's life was the dark angel of law, Roy Cohn. Cohn's legal past was nefariously marked by being an effective and ruthless prosecutor at the controversial espionage trial of Julius and Ethel Rosenberg, who later went to their deaths in the electric chair. Cohn was just twenty-three years old at the time. Later, at age twenty-six, he served as chief counsel to Senator Joseph McCarthy during the nightmarish, anti-Communist witch hunt Army-McCarthy hearings of 1954. Roy Cohn was adept at character assassination; after testifying, one witness committed suicide. Cohn's subsequent thirty-year law practice in Manhattan included a mixed medley of moguls and mobsters, ranging from New York Yankees owner George Steinbrenner, Aristotle Onassis, New

York's Cardinal Spellman, and the New York Catholic Diocese to Mafia chieftains John Gotti, Carmine "The Cigar" Galante, and Anthony "Fat Tony" Salerno.

A 2017 *Vanity Fair* article opined:

> *Who did not know Roy Cohn's backstory, even in 1980? Cohn—whose great-uncle had founded Lionel, the toy-train company—grew up as an only child, doted on by an overbearing mother who followed him to summer camp and lived with him until she died. Every night he was seated at his family's Park Avenue dinner table, which was an unofficial command post of the Favor Bank bosses who'd helped make his father, Al Cohn, a Bronx county judge, and later a State Supreme Court judge. During the Depression, Roy's uncle Bernard Marcus had been sent to prison in a bank-fraud case, and Roy's childhood was marked by visits to Sing Sing. By high school, Cohn was fixing a parking ticket or two for one of his teachers (Brenner, 2017).*

In *The Art of the Deal,* Trump described Cohn boasting that he had spent his entire life under indictment (for crimes including extortion, bribery, blackmail, perjury, obstruction of justice, securities, and tax fraud) but was never convicted. When Trump inquired to Cohn if he was actually guilty, Cohn responded, "What the hell do you think?" and just smiled. Trump has acknowledged that he never knew what that meant.

It is often stated in the media that Cohn was a "mentor" to Trump, but Trump always insisted that coveted appellation applied only to his father and Reverend Peale. For Trump, Cohn was "just a lawyer, a very good lawyer" (Kranish and Fisher, 2016). Cohn had several traits that Donald Trump valued, and first among them was loyalty. "He was a truly loyal guy—it was a matter of honor with him…you could count on him to go to bat for you, even if he privately disagreed with your view, and even if defending you wasn't necessarily the best thing for him. He was never two-faced." Added to loyalty was brilliance (Cohn graduated Columbia Law School at age twenty) and toughness.

> *Cohn possessed of a keen intellect…could keep a jury spellbound. When he was indicted for bribery, in 1969, his lawyer suffered a heart attack near the end of the trial. Cohn deftly stepped in and did a seven-hour closing argument—never once referring to a notepad. He was acquitted. 'I don't want to know what the law is,' he famously said, 'I want to know who the judge is' (Brenner, 2017).*

In 1973, at age twenty-seven, Trump first met Cohn one evening at a private Manhattan nightspot, Le Club. Amiably chatting, he shared with Cohn that Trump Management was being sued by the Department of Justice for housing discrimination. Trump was taken aback and impressed with Cohn's response: "My view is tell them to go to hell and fight the thing in court… [make them try and prove it]" (Trump and Schwartz, 1987). This stance of "admit nothing and deny everything" "claim victory, sue, and counter-sue," as well as "swiftly exercise fear-provoking threats of suits and counter-suits," became Trump's legal modus operandi. Donald had already heard the clarion call of "never admit defeat," from his mentor Reverend Peale. Cohn was, in a sense, preaching to the choir. But long before Cohn, even Peale had his germinating words fall on fertile ground. Recall that Donald from childhood was "aggressive" (not "mischievous"), and as a high school athlete was fiercely competitive. These teachers offered their skills to a willing learner.

Cohn was Trump's attack dog until his death from AIDS in 1986. In 1980 Cohn told *Vanity Fair* reporter Marie Brenner, "Donald calls me 15-20 times a day...He is always asking, what is the status of this, and that?" It was also Cohn who introduced Trump to stringent pre-nuptial agreements (to Ivana's surprise and shock), a policy he implemented in his two subsequent marriages.

Peale was a valued mentor who offered a spiritual, philosophical, psychological framework for Trump. It named Trump's natural tendencies, stamped them as laudable and desirable, even spiritual. Cohn offered a legal defense that featured a strong offense. It is a legal form of the "anchoring bias" previously outlined by Cernovich, and gives Trump room to negotiate from strength of assumed victory rather than closed-book defeat. The crushing political defeat of the US/Mexican wall to end the January 2018 government shutdown was confidently presented in the White House Rose Garden (appropriately named for the metaphorical spectacles about to be employed) as a strategic opportunity. There is no doubt Roy Cohn would smilingly approve. Unlike Roy Cohn, President Trump's "anchoring bias" can shift when strategically pragmatic; he is not locked into it as a matter of principal, but more as a matter of strategy. Naturally this ease of shifting dismays President Trump's critics, especially when the starting point seemed blatantly untrue and is not apologized for in the shift, but for President Trump it is probably applying his pragmatic brand of business negotiations to Washington politics. So, with opening of diplomatic channels, President Trump can easily shift from threatening North Korea with annihilation to protestations of love for its president.

A Few Longstanding Friendships

I've singled out Thomas J. Barrack Jr. as a prime example of Trump's openness to hearing different opinions, and it goes without saying that he is hardly the only person that Trump is in touch with. There are others outside the government whom he calls and some who call him. Many of these same people may be seen at Mar-a-Largo, which serves a similar function as the telephone in the White House bedroom; it is a place to meet, mingle, and gauge the temperature of opinion beyond Washington. But there are only a few, longstanding, trusted friends like Tom Barrack.

One is Richard LeFrak, who has known Trump for over forty years and shares with Trump a similar career in New York real estate. Unique to this friendship is the years of friendship both their fathers had with each other. Richard's father, Samuel J. LeFrak, was an early real estate innovator in New York. Richard LeFrak now manages a real estate empire that stretches coast-to-coast. LeFrak has tellingly said of Trump: "Donald has some friends like me, but he's much more of a homebody than you'd think. He's very gregarious and has lots of acquaintances. But people that he's close to? Not so many.... If we're both in Florida, Donald might call and say, 'Come have dinner at Mar-a-Lago'...But if I tell him, 'Why don't you come down to Miami,' he might say yes, but he probably won't do it. He's very much a creature of habit. He doesn't like to leave his own environment."

LeFrak, good friend that he is, grasps the nature of Trump's "private self." Of Trump's persona, LeFrak has also said: "He's the kind of guy who likes throwing hand grenades in the room. There's a lot of intensity and energy, a lot of publicity and other stuff. Being friends with Trump is like being friends with a hurricane" (Feuer, 2016). Interestingly, to LeFrak whom Trump sees as one of his closest friends, Trump has revealed both sides of his personality—the persona and the private self—a true sign of the tightness of their bond.

Another friend of over thirty years and often named by Trump as one of his closest friends is the successful businessman Howard Lorber, who is the chief executive of Vector Group, a holding company that's ventured into real estate and tobacco. One of his investments known best to New Yorkers is ironically one of his smaller investments; he owns Nathan's Famous, the hot dog icon of the city. Of note, the first "Nathan's" was in Brooklyn's Coney Island in 1916, the site of Fred Trump's earliest building (and advertising) successes. Lorber was an economic adviser to Trump's presidential campaign, a significant fundraiser for Trump (including raising funds for his 2020 campaign) and was named by President Trump as chairman of the U.S. Holocaust Memorial Council. During a CNBC interview

Lorber was asked about Donald Trump's temperament, leading him to enthusiastically describe Trump and Melania as "warm" people that on innumerable occasions have telephoned or left caring messages to inquire routinely after Lorber and his family. When asked if Trump is racist, Lorber vigorously replied: "No! After almost 35 years of knowing him, I never heard a prejudiced word come out of his mouth, not about color, race, religion, sexuality, nothing! He's prejudiced against only one type of person, the person who attacks him first.... [Asked if Trump listens... Lorber laughs! and adds] He listens! [Lorber laughed again] He is a questioner, he asks questions, filters things, and then makes his own decisions" (Frank, October 2016), (Frank, November 2016). This cognitive style of organizing understanding through questioning has a long history, as Trump has recounted: "Not too long ago I received a letter from my kindergarten teacher. It was a big surprise for me to find that in one of those piles of letters [I receive]. She mentioned that what she remembered most clearly about me is that I never stopped asking questions. I was the most inquisitive student she had ever had. I wrote back to her that some things never change—I still ask a lot of questions—but that my curiosity and sense of discovery has served me well" (Trump and McIver, 2008).

There is also a significant female, longtime friend worthy of mention and that is Linda McMahon, who, along with her husband, founded what is now World Wrestling Entertainment. Her husband, Vince McMahon, challenged Donald Trump in 1988 to a Wrestlemania IV celebrity match called *The Battle of the Billionaires.* Donald beat Vince and got to shave Vince's vaunted hair in the ring to the wild approval of the crowded arena. The McMahons became weighty donors to Trump's political campaigns and charities. Linda McMahon has said: "Once he's your friend, he is loyal to the end." Trump named Linda McMahon head of the Small Business Administration and she served in that position until 2019 (Jaffe, 2017).

The front office at The White House may be in rotational turmoil, as President Trump finds his way in Washington, but his capacity for longterm, stable relationships is unquestionably present. In his new political world this capacity will become increasingly evident as time goes on. In addition, one can check the media accounts of visitors to Mar-a-Largo, where one can find a wide and changing swarth of American political, business, entertainment, sports, and government life who meet and engage Trump.

More Friends and Acquaintances

Although one often reads of President Donald Trump's enduring friendships with other powerhouses of American accomplishment, such as Rudy Giuliani, the former Mayor of New York; Stephen Schwarzman, CEO of Blackstone Group; Robert Kraft, owner of The New England Patriots; or Newt Gingrich, former Speaker of the United States House of Representatives, there are lower profile friendships that reveal a softer, empathic side of Trump.

While an electric performer, Michael Jackson was painfully shy in off-stage, personal interaction. Donald Trump was sensitive to this side of Jackson, always tactful and respectful, as well as openly warm. They became, in Trump's words, "good friends." Jackson accepted Trump's invitation to Mar-a-Largo for Jackson's honeymoon with his new wife, Lisa Marie Presley. Michael Jackson never knew that Trump had emptied all the rooms and public areas near them to guarantee their privacy. Trump kept their space secluded. The new couple said their stay was magical.

"Iron" Mike Tyson is hardly thought of as a fragile, vulnerable individual. But prior to his current excellent marriage, in earlier years, his romantic life and finances were repeated calamities. When Mike Tyson was sentenced to prison one of his first telephone calls was to his friend, Donald Trump. Trump felt a devotion to the beaten-down Tyson as he faced prison, and went to great lengths to get a substitute sentence for him, one that avoided prison and offered community service. It was refused. Perhaps as payment to Trump for financial assistance during one of Tyson's bouts with financial disaster, a boxing championship belt hung in the Trump Tower office.

Similar friendships were developed by Trump with the elderly group of gardeners when he acquired Mar-a-Largo. Many of the gardeners were at the estate from its inception and were now in their seventies. He kept them all on in their usual capacities. One became ill, and after hospitalization, Trump put him up gratis at Mar-a-Largo for his entire recovery. A similar soft side of Trump was visible with Jennifer Hudson after the tragic murders of her mother and brother in 2008. Trump arranged a hotel suite at the Trump International Hotel Tower gratis for Hudson and her family (Evon, 2017). In 2013, Trump was moved by a news story of a bus driver named Darnell Barton who talked a woman down from jumping off a bridge and sent him a check for $10,000. His note to the driver read, "Although I know to you it was just a warm-hearted first response to a dangerous situation, your quick thinking resulted in a life being saved, and for that you should be rewarded" (Evon, 2017).

These anecdotes are not usually heard from Trump's personae, either as campaigner or president. But they are nonetheless part of who he is, and many more could be told.

Fantasy Friends

In early life Donald Trump imagined he might either be a builder or a baseball player. At age twelve, at Kew-Forest School in Queens, Donald composed an ode to baseball for his school yearbook, writing, "I like to hear the crowd give cheers, so loud and noisy to my ears. When the score is 5-5, I feel like I could cry. And when they get another run, I feel like I could die. Then the catcher makes an error, not a bit like Yogi Berra. The game is over and we say tomorrow is another day" (Schwartzman and Miller, 2016).

Through all of military school, Trump was an outstanding, award-winning athlete in several sports, rising to captain of the baseball team. He loved playing catcher most of all. Trump the catcher was described by teammates as rugged behind the plate. Foul balls blasted off his mask and wild pitches saved with his chest protector. A superb hitter, he was concordantly fierce on the base paths. Colleges dangled sports scholarships.

Two of New York City's most beloved sports figures were Yogi Berra of the New York Yankees and Roy "Campy" Campanella of the Brooklyn Dodgers, both of whom were iron-men catchers.

Berra and Campanella were idols of Trump's whom he adored above all other sports figures. Berra and Campanella were loved and respected by teammates and fans alike. They were earthy, good-humored, affectionate, splendid ballplayers, endowed with endless endurance and energy. As catchers, they were detail players who were always in the action. Their personalities enthralled the everyday fan as well as aficionados. Reporters relished them. Since they also both played in an era when players often spent their whole major league careers with one team—as these two did—they probably also aroused young Trump's admiration for their loyalty.

In Yogi and Campy we see a Rorschach slice of Trump's mind, his values and goals. To what degree and in what form he actualized these fantasized longings, I have partially described. But, particularly, Trump excelled as both a star and a team player, a captain. It is this dual capacity that is essential in a president who must navigate between his goals and the goals of those around him. It is important to know that this duality is inherent to Trump's nature.

You Can't Judge a Person by their Persona

For over fifty years Donald Trump has been shaping his persona as his personal brand. It started as a business persona, then added an entertainment persona, followed by a campaign persona. We're now witnessing the molding of a presidential persona. They are all related and grow out of the same personality substrates. They are not add-ons, but rather elaborations.

Many speculate that President Trump is changing throughout the presidency (Baker, 2017), but that is doubtful. Essentially, what we see are seventy-two-year-old wines in new White House bottles—and after all, that is what he promised.

CHAPTER

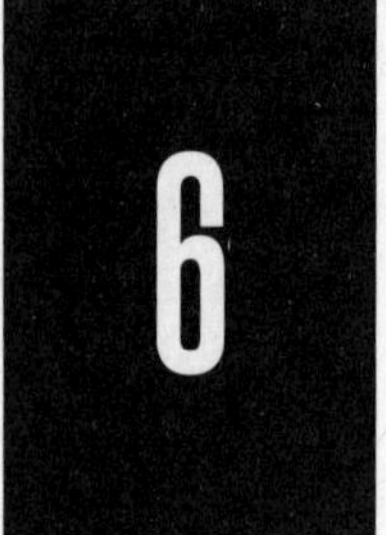

SUBSTANCE, STYLE, AND SUITABILITY FOR PRESIDENTIAL LEADERSHIP

A Leader's Mark

What can we see in the substance of President Trump's goals, achievements, and style of work? Does this profile add up to suitability for presidential leadership? Where does his distinctive personality fit into the profound demands of presidential office? How does he compare to the historical record of those who struggled with presidential challenges of the past?

Richard Nixon said that the mark of a leader "is whether he can give history a nudge" (Osnos, 2018). Giving "history a nudge" captures what I believe will be Trump's mark on the history of American presidencies and our nation. What this "nudge" will consist of, only time can judge, but there are several possible areas:

- Peace with North Korea
- An Israeli-Palestinian peace
- An end to the Saudi-Yemen war
- China's growing international menacing hegemony, formerly unconfronted, challenged and rebalanced
- Iran realigned with consequent Middle East stabilization
- A shift in the federal judiciary toward conservatism
- America remaining the world's primary power
- America spared the civil upheavals of Europe induced by uncontrolled immigration
- A Mexican-American wall bringing positive social and economic changes
- Splintering of the Democratic and Republican parties leading to a parliamentarian-like coalition government
- Stunning "supply-side" economic success due to tax cuts

Surprisingly, I found some support for my speculation in *The Boston Globe* of all places. The *Globe* has been consistently anti-Trump. Despite that, the op-ed was boldly titled, "Trump is breaking all the rules, and that could be great for America" (Ferguson, 2018). Speaking as a future historian, the editorial states:

> *President Trump had no experience of foreign affairs, but he soon grasped how disastrously his predecessor had bungled the North Korean nuclear threat. He applied sustained pressure on Pyongyang, directly through new UN-mandated sanctions, and indirectly by menacing China with threats of military action or a trade war.... In March 2018, he stepped up the pressure by announcing new tariffs on steel and aluminum imports. These tariffs would have hurt America's allies more than China, but Beijing got the message. Xi Jinping was well aware a trade war directed by the US against China would hurt China much more than the United States, potentially reducing Chinese exports to America by up to 20 percent. The president's critics were stunned by the subsequent US-North Korean Strategic Arms Limitation Treaty, signed in Pyongyang in 2019, and utterly dumbfounded by the 2020 Chinese-American Trade Agreement, which committed China to eliminate the bilateral trade deficit by the end of his second presidential term.*

Speculation about Trump's future image aside, a 2018 Gallup Poll found the majority of Americans call President Trump "intelligent, strong, and a decisive leader." For the 1,520 adults surveyed June 1–13, 2018, 58 percent said they think Trump "is intelligent," while 51 percent said he "is a strong and decisive leader" and 50 percent said he "can bring about the changes this country needs" (Cochran, 2018). Should Trump go on to achieve any of the feats listed, voter confidence will grow even further.

An Outsized Personality

CNBC veteran White House reporter Keith Koffler has described the personality and psychology of President Trump as ideally fitted for the international crises of our age.

> *Not too long ago, the struggles among great nations were defined by ideology, as democracy and communism competed for allegiance around the world. During that age, a relatively non-ideological, nonintellectual man like Trump might have had trouble understanding the thinking animating Russian and Chinese communists, hampering his ability to confront them. But with realpolitik and raw ambition supreme, Trump is the man for this current age of crisis. The president will have no problem understanding the motivations of Kim and the other tyrants he faces, including Russian President Vladimir Putin, newly anointed Chinese President-for-Life Xi Jingping and Iranian supreme leader Ayatollah Ali Khamenei. And Trump has the outsized strength of personality to combat them—unlike any of his rivals in the 2016 presidential election (Koffler, 2018).*

Turning standard anti-Trump criticism on its head, Koffler thinks it is exactly Trump's ruthless business nature that "might just be brutal and dark enough to stand his ground against [tyrants] and counter their own ruthless agendas." Koffler ironically acknowledges that it is exactly the qualities he personally distains in President Trump's psychology that are best suited to ensure America's safety. As an astute reviewer of presidential scholar Doris Kearns Goodwin's recent book on presidential leadership determined: "No one turns up in the White House by accident, even 'accidental presidents' like Harry Truman" (Shribman, 2018).

On the list, it's Trump's extraordinary economic accomplishments that are least likely to be felt as a "nudge." As historian Richard Reeves observed, "Nobody remembers whether Abraham Lincoln or Franklin D. Roosevelt or John F. Kennedy or Ronald Reagan balanced the budget" (Reeves, 2012).

Notice, however, that several of Trump's possible "nudges" on that list stem from solving crises, such as the threats of nuclear destruction, isolation, and war. Most historians agree that many of the great presidents earned that title during times of war (such as Polk, Lincoln, Wilson, FDR, Truman, and Eisenhower), or at times of an acute national crisis (such as JFK and the Cuban Missile Crisis). The caveat to this is that the president must be fighting a winning war to earn the title of "greatness." It can't be slow bleeding stalemates, national humiliations, and nation dividing frustrations like Vietnam, Iraq, and Afghanistan. These latter conflicts that resulted in unjustified human suffering, staggering financial cost, as well as failed international policies, were ingredients in the recipe that provided Trump with a vision: "Make America Great Again."

Transactional and Transformational Leadership

Reputable studies on leadership outline two major styles of leading: transactional and transformational (Odumeru and Ogbonna, 2013). Transactional leaders tend to work within the organizational culture and are competent during times of crisis because they default toward maintaining a status quo, often appealing to the individual interests of people through reward and punishment. Transformational leaders lead through vision. They are goal-oriented leaders who wish to change the culture at large and status quo. Their focus prioritizes group needs above individual needs. Our greatest presidents led with a vision and a goal. There was George Washington's federal union, Andrew Jackson's democracy for the people, Abe Lincoln's union and liberty, and Franklin Delano Roosevelt's social security and freedom through war. All fought a status quo; they were transformational.

The breadth of significant transformation is so formative, it exceeds the times in which the upending, disruptive changes were introduced. In her book *Leadership in Turbulent Times*, renowned historian Doris Kearns Goodwin pointed out in referencing Abraham Lincoln, Theodore Roosevelt, FDR, and Lyndon B. Johnson that "their paths were anything but certain.... Their stories abound in confusion, hope, failure and fear.... They are among the most compelling figures in our national story. Their lessons are among the most important as we plot our future" (Shribman, 2018). With transformational leadership, present is prologue.

Although I am not yet placing Donald Trump in the category of great presidents (because history will be his judge, as it is for every president), it's clear that his style of leadership is transformational. Trump's entire election platform was summarized in one simple slogan, "Make America Great Again." Trump portrayed Washington D.C. as a swamp in need of draining. The swamp represented a political elite that forgot the America that Trump remembered, and a Republican Party that had lost its way. Poor border control endangered national security and shoddy overseas entanglements threatened both safety and the economy. The rescue psychology of Trump's campaign vision is remarkably similar to the psychology that marked his most successful and disruptive real estate ventures in Manhattan.

Creative Disruption

As I outlined in "The Person and the Persona," in Trump's formative real estate ventures he disrupted the real estate status quo both in concept and in execution. It's worth again applying the archetype conceptions of Trump's favorite psychologist, Carl Jung, to outline this behavioral theme as it courses through Trump's real estate life until the presidency.

For the sake of understanding, Trump's psychological archetypes need a recap. Through all of Trump's writings there runs a theme of builder as "hero" (a major archetype, like Hercules). His real estate projects are envisioned as restoring decayed entities (such as the Commodore and surrounding Times Square neighborhood), generating life (acres of Manhattan's Westside Penn Central Railroad Yards laying fallow), awakening potential (Trump Tower), bringing innovative vision to stagnant real estate blindness (40 Wall Street reinvented), rescuing New York City from bureaucracy (Central Park Wollman Skating Rink), and restoring a "beat-up, overgrown Rembrandt" (Mar-a-Largo). Most of Trump's projects involved Herculean challenges—economic, political, architectural, and cultural. The odds were against Trump, as a builder, a campaigner, and now as president. I think he loves it—the scrapper athlete of his youth continuously emerges as challenger to take on the establishment.

In Trump's view, what was transformative for Manhattan's decayed Forty-Second Street or inadequately developed Fifth Avenue and Fifty-Sixth Street is now transposed to the hobbled nation—and due to America's influence, to the world. It may sound unrealistically large, but Trump is the president of the most powerful nation in the world. He had, and has, a large vision and a goal (making America great again) that resonates with his base. Between the vision and its goal, however, is a pathway—and the devil is in the details.

The Power to Persuade

Deep understanding is reflected in concise explanations. One of the leading political analysts of the twentieth century, Richard Neustadt deftly summarized his research into presidential power as "the power to persuade" (Neustadt, 1990). Persuasion and bargaining are the means that presidents use to implement policy. And this persuasive power must always be looking down the road, around the corner, to the next point of persuasion and bargaining. Power cannot be dissipated on the present moment; it must always be geared toward the acquisition of future power. Favors traded now imply favors in the future. It is the possession of bargaining chips that gives persuasive power, and if used correctly, increases power. If this conception sounds Machiavellian, then you definitely understand Neustadt.

Neustadt distinguishes persuasive power from the powers authorized to the president by the constitution. Persuasive power is the power to influence others. President Truman, envisioning General Eisenhower coming into presidential office, said, "He'll sit here [at the president's desk]...and he'll say, 'Do this! Do that!' And nothing will happen. Poor Ike—It won't be like the Army. He'll find it frustrating." Earlier, Truman had remarked, "I sit here all day trying to persuade people to do the things they ought to have sense enough to do without my persuading them.... That's all the powers of the President amount to" (Neustadt, 1990).

Loyalty and Power

It was only in reading Neustadt that I gleaned the importance of Donald Trump's lifelong insistence on "loyalty" as a first order requirement in relationships with people, most of whom were business associates, workers, and now, members of the administration. Trump has unequivocally stated: "I value loyalty above everything else—more than brains, more than drive, and more than energy" (Trump and Zanker, 2007). For Trump, family loyalty is the gold standard, against which all others are measured.

Loyalty means you can be sure of power and that your actions will not negate your power due to the assurance of loyalty. With Trump, loyalty assures power.

Of course, nothing is black or white, and if Trump were to engage in excessively egregious actions that no one could be loyal to, out would go his power. For example, the evangelicals forgive much in his unevangelical behavior, but if he were to renounce belief in God, it would probably be the end of their support. Although, I guess that even then, some evangelicals would remain loyal, waiting for his repentance. But it is part of his political wiliness that he seems to go up to a red line, but not go far enough to alienate his supporters. Indeed, the media are always astounded that regardless of seeming scandal—sexual impropriety, blurred ethical boundaries, mixing personal business with government business, questions of nepotism, outrageous tweets, Trump's support remains solid with his base. They are loyal.

Loyalty and Chaos

The psychological reliance on loyalty has contributed to the chaos of Trump's White House administration. We read repeatedly of the record number of turnovers of positions in the administration, some for scandal, some for inadequacy, but mostly for lack of loyalty. Excessive disagreement is intolerable to Trump, and perhaps it should be so, because how can one accomplish the goals of a vision if the pathway is constantly blocked. A stark example is the former Secretary of State, Rex Tillerson, who set many roadblocks to Trump's vision. They differed sharply, and usually publicly, on Iran, North Korea, Israel, Saudi Arabia-Qatar, and Russia.

In New York, Trump lived in a circumscribed world, a world he had occupied since childhood. Builders, tradespeople, local union bosses, politicians—these were all household names to him for a lifetime, and he is seventy-two. Out of hundreds of contractors, he could name only a handful he could trust. Washington is a foreign land of politics without the same reliable, hands-on, personal familiarity he had with business. Trump's style of hiring and firing is somewhat instinctive in nature; he calls it "chemistry." In choosing Mike Pompeo to succeed Rex Tillerson, Trump said, "We have a very good relationship, for whatever reason, chemistry, whatever it is—why do people get along? I've always, right from the beginning, from day one, I've gotten along well with Mike Pompeo" (Landler, Haberman, Gardiner, 2018). Trump will accept a candidate well vetted by others, and whom he does not know personally, but once he smells disloyalty, it is the emotional acid test, and the person will be let go. This style is new to Washington, shocking to those who fear an inbred cabal of über-hawks (Wright, 2018), but whether it ultimately prevents Trump's vision reaching its goal, remains to be seen.

Persuasion Through Communication

Another form of persuasion in the pursuit of power is communication. FDR bypassed Congress with radio "fireside chats." Reagan was known as "the great communicator." Meanwhile, Trump speaks most directly to the public through Twitter. Trump's reliance on going to the people directly perhaps stems from his lack of longtime loyal ties among the political elite of Congress and the deep administrative bureaucracy (the "Fourth Estate" of government). Plus, the lack of cohesion in either the Republican Party or the Democratic Party, adds to the stunting complication of using bargaining as a form of persuasion; splintering of political forces splinters the leverage of persuasion.

By "going public," Trump seeks to augment his persuasive power outside of Congress and the wider administration. He has relied on several public formats: televised meetings with members of Congress, group rallies, and robust, daily tweeting sessions. He also enjoys TV appearances with favored newscasters like Sean Hannity or Judge Jeanine Pirro.

Unscripted, unrehearsed, publicly televised White House meetings are novel innovations for the presidency. They showcase President Trump with a revolving cast of congressional members. It allows direct questioning, a back and forth repartee, and the spontaneity of a political setting engages home viewers. For example, on one broadcast, sitting beside Trump was a usual political nemesis, Senator Diane Feinstein (D-CA). When President Trump proffered remarks favorable to her view of gun control, she broke into warm smiles. The sudden melting of the usual ice between them broadcast to the nation a compromising, negotiable, president—one who looked ready to bargain. Whether this moment led to her desirable legislative hopes is not the point (which it did not), but rather that different sides of Trump were viewed by the nation. And, from Trump's point of view, the media did not filter it.

There are risks to "going public," and, of course, Trump is a risk taker par excellence! "Going public" does not contain the substantial, nitty-gritty details of bargaining, lacks the mutual advantages of striking a bargain, it runs the risk of hardening positions and making bargaining harder, and it undermines the authority of Congress, possibly inciting resentment among members. Further, it risks public embarrassment when the stance taken is defeated, either at the ballot box (when a supported candidate suffers defeat) or in Congress (Kernell, 2007). Certainly, the disastrous 2018–2019 government shutdown was an example of a failure of "going public." Trump's televised appeals and tweets to the nation failed to match the persuasive power of behind-the-scenes, well-crafted, bargaining of his political opponents.

A variant of Trump's direct-to-the-people style of persuasion is his daily and frequent use of the telephone. Many longtime senators and House members state they never had such easy telephone access to the president in former administrations. President Trump's use of the telephone is strikingly new. Trump picks up calls directly, or calls are routed swiftly through the White House director of Oval Office operations, or directly via the White House switchboard. The ease of phone communication goes both ways, as Trump usually initiates calls without warning. Senate Majority Leader Mitch McConnell was once telephoned while attending a baseball game. Senator Joe Manchin III (D-WV) was skyping with a group of high school students. Senator James M. Inhofe (R-OK) was chopping wood with his grandson (Kim and Dorsey, 2019). Mark Leibovich, in *The New York Times*, reported that a few hours prior to President Trump's 2019 State of the Union address he called Senator

Lindsey Graham asking: "Should I go conciliatory or to-hell-with-it? What kind of tone should I take?" Lindsey shared with the reporter that "I have never been called this much by a president in my life." Leibovich continued: "[Lindsey's] tone reflected a mixture of amazement and amusement, with perhaps a dash of awe. 'It's weird, and it's flattering, and it creates some opportunity. It also creates some pressure.'" Leibovich's capture of "a dash of awe" particularly caught my attention since it is the subject of this book's last chapter, "Insufficient Awe."

Again, we see the rerouting of Trump's business style adapting to Washington. At Trump Tower his two major filterers of life, Norma Foerderer and Rhona Graff, fielded several hundred telephone calls a week. Trump was often on the telephone all day long as people wandered in and out of his always open-door office. At the White House, however, Trump moves into personal-self mode as these telephone calls are mostly conducted during his extensive "executive time," a time sequestered in his White House bedroom, which usually begins around 6 PM. At Trump Tower he focused on as many building details as humanly possible. This same obsessive style is reflected in many congressional members indicating that they trusted a presidential telephone conversation more than information obtained from a White House aide, since it seemed that only Trump could be trusted to speak for Trump (Kim and Dorsey, 2019). Trump's calls are unpredictable in content, ranging from requests for feedback about his agendas, responding to seeing them on TV, hunting for ideas, or just "to chat."

The Mantle of Andrew Jackson

Although Trump heralded himself as an outsider, he has draped an insider's mantle over his psychological shoulders, a robust identification with the seventh POTUS, Andrew Jackson. In addition to proudly placing Jackson's portrait in the Oval Office, Trump visited his home in Tennessee shortly after inauguration (Glaser, 2018). For Trump, identification with Jackson grants Trump entry to the halls of unquestioned, historical insiders.

Like Jackson, Trump is a populist—the voice of forgotten, disenfranchised Americans. Jackson leaned on his view that the president was the only officer of government elected by all the people and it was his responsibility to carry out their will (Johannsen, 1999). Trump echoes the same mandate, his campaign promises. Jackson abhorred overseas entanglements, favored tariffs, and railed against the established Washington elite. Both brought their own "outside elite" to Washington. Both deplored excessive federal regulation and court mandated laws over their programs.

Trump's populist nature is reflected in his pre-White House living style. He was not cloistered in a gated estate in the countryside. Trump Tower is smack in the middle of dense New York City. Although Trump has his home on the top three floors of Trump Tower, the bottom half of the building is a warren of bustling businesses, shops. and restaurants, always filled with people. The several stories high entry atrium is a major tourist attraction, a public thoroughfare; and it was from here that Trump chose to announce his run for the presidency. Similarly, Mar-a-Lago may be an expensive country club, but unlike many corners of Palm Beach it is open to all, regardless of ethnicity, gender, sexual orientation, or religion. Both anchors of living imbedded the Trump persona in an endless, stimulating sea of people.

Although Trump has never compared their communication techniques, it is fascinating that in Jackson's time, like Trump, Jackson was an innovator in political marketing, especially with newspapers (again, shades of *Citizen Kane*!). Jackson subscribed to as many as seventeen newspapers, which has parallels to Trump's ceaseless surfing of TV news. Jackson personally influenced newspaper articles and courted news editors (analogous to Trump's tireless tweeting), and advanced a new, pro-Jackson Washington newspaper, *United States Telegraph*—Jackson's own Fox News network, as it were (Hughes, 1828) (Inskeep, 2016).

Less publicly vaunted was the ease with which Jackson's tender self-esteem felt wounded and dishonored. Jackson is reputed to have fought as many as one hundred duels, killing three men. He's said to have carried embedded bullets from those encounters for the rest of his life (Klein, March 2017). Trump is a bit more civilized; he tweets and fires people.

James Parton, who wrote one of the early, respected biographies of Andrew Jackson, penned a summary of Jackson's conflicting character traits that bear great similarity to descriptions leveled at Trump:

> *Andrew Jackson, I am given to understand, was a patriot and a traitor. He was one of the greatest generals, and wholly ignorant of the art of war. A brilliant writer, elegant, eloquent, without being*

> *able to compose a correct sentence or spell words of four syllables. The first of statesmen, he never devised, he never framed, a measure. He was the most candid of men, and was capable of the most profound dissimulation. A most law-defying law-obeying citizen. A stickler for discipline, he never hesitated to disobey his superior. A democratic autocrat. An urbane savage. An atrocious saint (Parton, 1860).*

Trump's energizing psychological identification with President Jackson, an outsized, controversial personality—Thomas Jefferson famously referred to Andrew Jackson as a "dangerous man"—leads us to the frequently debated issue by his political opponents of Trump's mental health.

A Circus of Diagnoses

Perhaps it is a reflection of the largeness of Donald Trump's personality and the diverse paths his life has taken, that so many psychiatric diagnoses have been thrown in his direction: narcissistic personality disorder, malignant narcissism, narcissistic alexithymia, bi-polar disorder, hypomanic temperament, delusional disorder, paranoid, sociopath/psychopath, senile dementia, extreme hedonism, histrionic personality disorder, impulse disorder, attention deficit/ hyperactivity disorder (ADHD), dyslexia, and even normality in Donald Trump's hands is transmogrified—pathologized—as "malignant normality" (like the Nazi doctors) (Lee, 2017).

Although these diagnoses are usually made by qualified professionals, even more qualified and accomplished professionals have refuted such claims with ease and determined that President Trump does not demonstrate any diagnosable mental illnesses (Begley, 2017). In fact, the very author of psychiatry's *Diagnostic and Statistical Manual of Mental Disorders* (DSM) section on narcissistic personality disorder, Allen Frances M.D., stated that Trump does not demonstrate such a disorder, and even further, concluded that Trump is not mentally ill (Frances, 2017). Professor Frances is unequivocal: "Trump doesn't meet DSM criteria [for any mental disorder]…. I wrote the criteria and should know how they are meant to be applied: Personality disorder requires the presence of clinically significant distress and/or impairment" (Begley, 2017). Furthermore, in January 2017, the results of President Trump's annual medical exam found him physically healthy, not impaired cognitively, and made no recommendations for a psychiatric consultation (Shear and Altman, 2017). After examination by eleven medical specialists, a similar clean bill of health was delivered in 2019 (Gearan, 2019). The exception to this recent excellent health report was a weight gain that now qualifies the president for a diagnosis of obesity (Associated Press, 2019).

For many decades The American Psychiatric Association has required that persons diagnosed as mentally ill have two essential characteristics: (1) significant disturbances of emotion, belief, or behavior, and (2) cause the person to suffer clinically significant distress or impairment. President Trump is no different from who he was for over five decades as a businessman. Over his long life, I agree with President Trump's personal personality assessment: "I am…very stable" (his "genius" addition isn't essential to the description). Indeed, personality traits are stable over time, and the attainment of power may spotlight those traits. It is understandable that Trump's policies and even his behavior may not be to one's liking or political persuasion, but they are not reflective of mental illness.

A Sound Mind in a Sound Body

Psychiatric articles struggling to describe mental health are often marked by lists of early signs of mental disorder. Prime among these early warning signs are social withdrawal, mood disturbances, failure at work, domestic disruptions, sleep disorders, sharp increases or decreases in energy level, strange new behaviors, personal appearance, drug addiction or alcoholism, and cognitive decline and eating disorders.

Trump shows none of the foregoing warning signs of mental illness. He more closely fits the description of mental health given by the World Health Organization (WHO), which highlights mental health containing two key characteristics: "[Mental health is a] state of well-being in which the individual (1) realizes his or her own abilities, can cope with the normal stresses of life, can work productively and fruitfully, and (2) is able to make a contribution to his or her community." One aspect of Trump's general health that deserves special notice is his constitutional stamina, a quality desirable in a president. Through his whole adult life Trump has never required more than four to five hours of sleep a night, and he remains highly active and alert during waking hours. Corey Lewandowski, in his account of the presidential campaign, reports how absent daytime sleeping was in the candidate's regimen. Lewandowski recalled in over one thousand flight hours, he'd only seen Trump take a thirty-minute nap during long flights a handful of times. I have noticed the total lack of any medical report, either during the campaign or in all of the time post-election and through the White House presidency, in which Donald Trump was reported ill, having the sniffles, or needing a day off to rest. Trump's golf outings usually go eighteen holes, played vigorously, competitively, and frequently. Also noteworthy is Trump's lifelong, total abstinence from alcohol, smoking, and drug use. Apart from drinking twelve Diet Cokes a day, no other American president matches this triad of lifetime health habits.

In assessing fitness for the presidency, it is important to bear in mind that in a study of thirty-seven American presidents from 1776–1974, 50 percent qualified for having at least some form of mental illness, and yet performed remarkably well in their presidential roles. For example, James Madison and Abraham Lincoln suffered depression; Theodore Roosevelt and Lyndon B. Johnson were deemed bi-polar; Ulysses Grant and Richard Nixon suffered with alcoholism; and Ronald Reagan, dementia (Winch, 2016).

Psychiatry and Politics

The use of psychiatric diagnoses to express political disagreement is alarming. It is highly reminiscent of post-Stalin Soviet Russia. After Stalin, although the gulags were gone, political murder was replaced by the psychiatric "hospitalization" of political opponents. Massive bouts of electroconvulsive therapy and mind-numbing doses of psychotropic drugs were administered in prison-like psychiatric hospital conditions that reduced people to veritable zombies. After the fall of the Soviet Union, in 1991 during Russia's period of *perestroika* (rebuilding), I was part of an American group of psychiatrists invited to Russia to teach psychodynamic and psychoanalytic therapy—"talking therapy," which gives voice to taboo thoughts. These concepts and writings were illegal under the Soviets, punishable by time in the gulag. During repeated visits to Russia I continued to hear sad stories of the abusive use of psychiatry to squelch opposition in the former Soviet Union. Common in these painful remembrances were the misuse of psychotropic medications to drug and cognitively disable the victim's mental abilities and applying electroconvulsive therapy to obliterate memory and feelings. This current upsurge of psychiatric labeling—political psychiatric shaming—poses a threat to our democratic system, which relies on political rhetoric and votes to express opposition. Former Harvard Law School professor Alan Dershowitz, has stated, "The 25th Amendment would require, for mental incapacity, a major psychotic break. This is hope over reality. If we don't like someone's politics, we rail against him, we campaign against him; we don't use the psychiatric system against him. That's just dangerous" (Karni, 2018). Elsewhere, Dershowitz looked back at the 1964 presidential election between Democratic President Lyndon B. Johnson and Republican Senator Barry Goldwater:

> *I was shocked to read an article in FACT magazine, based on interviews with more than 1,000*

> *psychiatrists, which concluded that Goldwater was mentally unstable and psychologically unfit to be president. It was Lyndon Johnson whose personal fitness to hold the highest office I questioned. Barry Goldwater seemed emotionally stable with excellent personal characteristics, but highly questionable politics. The article was utterly unpersuasive, and in the end, I reluctantly voted for Lyndon Johnson. Barry Goldwater went back to the Senate, where he served with great distinction and high personal morality. Lyndon Johnson got us deeply into an unwinnable war that hurt our nation. The more than 1,000 psychiatrists, it turned out, were dead wrong in their diagnosis and predictions... They just didn't like his politics (Dershowitz, 2018).*

The *FACT* article had published psychiatric claims like: "It is...abundantly clear to me that he has never forgiven his father for being a Jew.... [Another concluded] The core of his paranoid personality is...his anality and latent homosexuality.... [And yet another wrote] I believe Goldwater has the same pathological make-up as Hitler, Castro, Stalin and other known schizophrenic leaders" (Resnick, 2017). The wide range of diagnoses applied to Senator Goldwater is remarkably similar to the aforementioned list of labels assigned to President Trump. These two gentlemen could never be mistaken one for the other, except perhaps for some similarities in politics.

Ironically, opponents of President Trump who insist on disqualifying the president as unsuitable for his role based on mental illness are losing an opportunity for presenting their own essential arguments. *The New England Journal of Medicine* reviewed the history of "medicalization and demedicalization" of diagnoses initially considered medical "diseases" (i.e., homosexuality, wrongly classified as a mental illness) and how the cultural prejudices surrounding the medicalization were thereby obscured or lost. These unscientific social biases were not challenged or publicly debated. The history of such medicalization reveals how much political and moral debates of the times were key to the creation of the diagnoses. These social, moral, political issues became highlighted only when the medicalized diagnosis was disproved and discarded, demedicalized. In other words, opponents of Trump who champion "medical" reasons for his removal from office, should stick to politics, as knotty, blurred, and anxiously controversial as those issues may be, they will be closer to real differences in policy. Plus, these political differences are more likely understandable to all citizens, not just mental health professions (Braslow and Messac, 2018).

Polk the Mendacious

Some wiser critics of Trump avoid speculating about his sanity, and focus on personality traits they deem problematic: boasting, arrogance, impulsiveness, distractibility, self-centeredness, volatility, among others. One that particularly vexes detractors is distortion of the truth, or out-and-out fabrication (Kessler, 2018). Yet, history suggests the assessment of such personality nuances evolves over time.

According to *The Washington Post* "fact checker," as of September 12, 2018, President Donald J. Trump had made over 5,000 false or misleading statements since obtaining the office of presidency. To emphasize the momentum of these fabrications, *The Washington Post* indicated that on Sept 7, 2018 in one day, in a time frame of 120 minutes in a Billings, Montana rally, President Trump set a new daily high, 74 "false or misleading claims" (Kessler, Rizzo and Kelly, 2018). The pattern of dubious claims has continued; for example, in the 2019 State of the Union address (Kessler, Rizzo and Kelly, 2019), and the doubtful suppositions he provided for the questionable declaration of a national state of emergency to fund the building of a border wall (Lybrand, 2019). At least one U.S. president parallels Trump in this regard.

James K. Polk was the eleventh president of the United States. During Polk's four-year term, almost one-third of our country was added to the map, linking us coast-to-coast, and fulfilling nineteenth century notions of America's manifest destiny. Through Polk's pursuit of war with Mexico, alternately threatening war or diplomacy with Britain, and outrageous manipulation of Congress, the United States obtained what is today: Texas, California, New Mexico, Arizona, Utah, Oregon, Washington, as well as additions to Kansas, Colorado, Oklahoma, Wyoming, and Montana. There were violently incensed, negative reactions to Polk's presidential actions.

Polk was widely reviled in his lifetime and long into the twentieth century. Robert Johannsen deftly describes Abraham Lincoln's dismay: "Lincoln nurtured his resentment for four years until 1848, when he finally exploded in fury over Polk's efforts to justify the war with Mexico.... Addressing the House of Representatives, he declared Polk was a liar...accused Polk with abusing the power of his office, contemptuously disregarding the Constitution, usurping the role of Congress and assuming the role of dictator.... [Polk's explanations were] 'the half-insane mumbling of a fever dream,' and Lincoln called down on Polk's head the wrath of God." At the other end of the nineteenth century, Ulysses S. Grant, in his memoirs, agreed with Lincoln, and maintained that the Civil War was God's punishment for Polk's sin. In repeated historical accounts, Polk was dubbed: "Polk the Mendacious" (Johannsen, 1999).

Polk, exhausted and ill, died within three months of leaving office in 1849. Upon the death of his widow in 1896, Polk's remarkable, detailed diary of his presidency was discovered. Pages yellowed, some, scribbled on with children's colored pencils, for fifty years it had lain in an attic box. In 1910 it was published in four volumes. The nation awoke to Polk's greatness. In the last seventy-five years of the twentieth century, increasingly positive opinions of Polk's presidency appeared.

President Harry Truman ranked Polk as one of the ten greatest presidents, and currently, Polk is usually ranked among the top ten to twelve presidents by many historians. Widely known as Young Hickory, Polk was determined to re-establish the program and policies of Andrew Jackson (nicknamed Old Hickory), and pursued Jacksonian-style, presidential power (Johannsen, 1999). I am sure Trump's identification with Andrew Jackson, and by implication, James Polk, is not lost on the reader. Just look at what happened to "Polk the Mendacious." History's verdict is as unpredictable and unknowable as the people who make it.

Sometimes, even in the short run there are dramatic, surprising shifts in political judgments. Take Lindsey Graham as an example. It was not long ago that Graham said of Trump, "I think he is a kook. I think he's crazy. I think he's unfit for office…He is a world class jackass…. [And] a race-baiting, xenophobic, religious bigot" (Baker and Haberman, 2018). Yet, recently the senator has become not only a privileged golf partner to President Trump, but now considers the president a political confidant, good friend, and supports many Trump policies. As reported in *The New York Times:* "Mr. Graham said he is the same old Lindsey, working with Mr. Trump when he can and disagreeing when he must. But he added of the president, 'being in his orbit, I think, has been good for me and good for him…. I enjoy his company…. I've spent more time talking to him than any president—all of them combined'" (Stolberg, 2018).

Just like with Polk, history cautions patience in judgment as it often smooths over fleeting Graham-like changes, and much remains to be judged. Whether President Trump's substance, style, and leadership builds on the past, is disruptively innovative, or fails, time will tell. If President Trump does give history a nudge, that nudge will not be measured by his mental state, healthy as it is, but rather, by its transformative consequences for America.

CHAPTER

7

NIAGARA FALLS

Room to Disagree

In the classic twentieth century comedy routine immortalized best by the comedy team of Bud Abbott and Lou Costello (or the Three Stooges), innocent, hapless Lou is in a small prison cell with a periodically delusional madman. Kind, unwitting Lou listens sympathetically to the initially calm cellmate's carefully related tale of woe, a love that suddenly, adulterously, unraveled. The forlorn cellmate describes searching the world for vengeance on the man who ruined his idyllic love, the brokenhearted sufferer finally finds the villain at Niagara Falls where he throttles the marital poacher within an inch of his life (which is why he is in prison). The mere mention of these toxic words, "Niagara Falls," transforms the morose composed storyteller—"Slowly I turned, step by step, inch by inch"—into a raging, delusional brute, throttling Lou Costello (or Curly Howard), until their desperate screams bring the madman back to sanity—only to have the whole sequence repeated over and over at the inadvertent mention of "Niagara Falls."

Despite being a Trump supporter myself, many of President Trump's attitudes and actions have a "Niagara Falls" impact on me, they induce an upsurge of exasperated anger with him. In an effort to help the reader understand that presenting Trump in a positive light does not automatically equal an endorsement of all his policies or behaviors, I want to outline my differences. My differences with President Trump do not suffice to erode my support of him.

Trump University

While I clearly believe that Donald Trump envisions himself as a guide, a mentor, a teacher, one who generously shares his accumulated knowledge—as repeatedly outlined in earlier chapters—I cannot reconcile myself to the inept, duplicitous venture of Trump University. An abundance of plausible testimony has described the failure of this supposed school to deliver what it promised, and promised at rather great tuition expense. I am at a complete loss at understanding, or finding a speculative rationale, for Donald Trump's ignorance of a project that he so fervently endorsed. Where were all the promised real estate experts? They were to be "hand-picked" by Trump; in testimony, he acknowledged never meeting any of them. Where was the unique course of instruction? Where were the promised personal appearances of Trump? I felt painful sadness looking at images of students taking "personal" photographs with a cardboard poster replica of Trump.

Although the courts decided in favor of the student plaintiffs' class action suit (Gerstein, 2017), supporting all their painful complaints, their financial retribution does not solve the ethical quandary. What was in Trump's mind at the inception of this misguided venture, during its ongoing failure, and now, as it is proved a fraudulent fiasco?

Nepotism

Thomas Jefferson warned: "The public will never be made to believe that an appointment of a relative is made on the ground of merit alone, uninfluenced by family views.... Nor can they see with approbation offices, the disposal of which they entrust to their Presidents for public purposes, divided out as family property."

In a cogent three-part series *The New York Times* editorial board traced the history of nepotism in the administrations of American presidents beginning with President John Adams, who appointed his son John Quincy Adams, a proven diplomat, as our first minister to Prussia (much to the dismay of Thomas Jefferson).

> *When critics said Franklin Roosevelt's appointment of his son James as White House secretary in 1937 [that led to administrative control over 18 federal agencies] allowed the young Roosevelt to enrich*

> *himself in the insurance business, in consult with his father he released five years of tax returns to prove otherwise [after continued journalistic criticism, he resigned from his post in November of 1938].... It was John F. Kennedy's appointment of his brother Robert as attorney general that led to the first anti-nepotism law in 1967. The nepotism law prohibited presidents and members of Congress from appointing or promoting relatives and spouses 'in or to a civilian position in the agency in which he is serving or over which he exercises jurisdiction or control'.... The Justice Department has cited that [Kennedy] law in a half-dozen legal opinions that prevented Presidents Richard Nixon, Jimmy Carter, Ronald Reagan and Barack Obama from appointing relatives to roles as minor as unpaid clerical assistant. (Editorial Board, Part 1, 2018).*

In a twist of irony, Trump benefited from the Clintons, who blurred the limits of acceptable nepotism. President Clinton appointed his wife as an unpaid advisor, a chairperson, to the task force on health care instead of as a paid formal government post. The unpaid, non-formal governmental post status bypassed a 1967 anti-nepotism statute. President Trump, in a similar Clintonian fashion, appointed Jared and Ivanka Kushner, as unpaid Senior White House Advisors, with a wide range of missions, domestic and foreign. Their qualifications for these missions are highly debatable, or more realistically, non-existent.

There is no limit to the unsupportable behavior from this couple as representatives of the United States government. At the 2017 G-20 meeting in Hamburg, Germany, Ivanka sat in for President Trump alongside Prime Minister Theresa May of England and Chancellor Merkel of Germany. As the last Seoul Olympics opened, President Trump tweeted: "My daughter, Ivanka, just arrived in South Korea. We cannot have a better, or smarter, person representing our country" (Editorial Board, Part 3, 2018). The last assertion is patently untrue, and while I have no qualms about fathers being blind to the extent of their progeny's abilities, I do have qualms about the president of the United States being in a similar paternal fog.

After representing the United States at the Seoul Olympics, and meeting with Kim Jung-un's sister, Ivanka was scheduled to meet with the visiting South Korean Foreign Minister Kang Kyung-wha. The United States was in the middle of preparations for Trump's meeting with Kim Jung-un; the issues were major ones—nuclear disarmament and war. What were her qualifications for these strategic meetings? None.

What demoralization does this behavior have on our State Department, the people who have dedicated long careers to these matters? As for Ivanka's domestic interests in women's issues, there has been neither significant congressional legislation nor government programs in those areas beyond sporadic conferences.

Additionally, Ivanka has shown no respect for boundaries between personal business and government business. *The New York Times* reported that on the day Ivanka and Jared met in China with the Chinese president, Xi Jinping, Ivanka Trump's company was granted three trademarks for the Chinese market. In public appearances, she has marketed her branded jewelry and businesses. To some extent, the former advent of John Kelly as Chief of Staff limited Ivanka's power. He had questioned her role, but even then, Kelly had little control over what happened outside that office (Trump's living quarters). Now that John Kelly is gone, the little control he had over her has gone with him.

A marker of Ivanka's political naivete and poor governmental judgment is her difficult-to-believe use of private emails for official government business, given her father's enduring haranguing of Hillary Clinton. Did Ivanka forget the chants of "lock her up!" in response to Hillary's egregious abuse of the law as Secretary of State? *The New Yorker* dubbed their review of this disturbing situation "The Entitled Hypocrisy of Ivanka Trump's Personal E-Mail Account." As part of the whitewashing of this violation of federal rules, Ivanka claimed ignorance of federal regulations. This is difficult to comprehend given the blaring media focus of her father's accusations against Hillary. And if ignorance is actually the case, what does this lackadaisical defense say about her capacity to be a senior advisor to the White House (Cassidy, 2018)?

Equally incredulous is Jared Kushner's role as diplomatic envoy to Mexico, China, and Canada, and as peace broker in the Middle East. Recent revelations document Kushner's family business as having a financial dependence on Chinese, Israeli, and Middle Eastern connections. *The New York Times* pointed out that "The Kushner family is scouring the globe for investors to shoulder billions in debt.... How handy then, that Jared Kushner who encumbered the family business (Kushner

Companies) with an overpriced, $1.8 billion skyscraper at 666 Fifth Avenue...is Mr. Trump's chief liaison with some two dozen nations, often operating outside formal guidance by the State Department or the National Security Council" (Editorial Board, Part 2, 2018). "Ethics watchdogs [had] previously lambasted the former tech entrepreneur and budding real estate magnate for not including one of his companies on a government financial disclosure form, in a move that allowed him to maintain a stake in the young startup while profiting from its explosive success during his transition to public service" (Riotta, 2017).

At one point in 2017, after much public criticism, Kushner's interim security clearance was downgraded from top secret to secret, meaning he no longer had access to the president's daily briefing. In May 2018, after several amendments to his security applications including supplying formerly missing material regarding foreign contacts (about one hundred foreign contacts were missing), he received permanent security clearance, once again giving him access to top secret material. Regardless, Kushner had long operated outside of State Department surveillance and had access to highly sensitive government material. Intercepted conversations between certain nations, including China and the United Arab Emirates, reveal Jared is considered "naïve" and easy to influence (Harris, Leonnig and Dawsey, 2018). Kushner's questionable security clearance has been again thrown into question by the revelation that President Trump intervened in the usual process of security clearance and ordered White House officials to obtain top-security clearance for his son-in-law. Trump previously denied having any part in the process of Kushner's security clearance. *The New York Times* alleged that with his order President Trump overruled the concerns and objections of intelligence officials, his then-chief of staff, John Kelly, and the White House counsel's office then led by Donald F. McGahn II. Given this contentious history, it is worrisome to think that Kushner is negotiating the peace process of the Middle East, some nations of which past Kushner business relationships remain in question (Haberman, Schmidt, Goldman and Karni, 2019).

"Kushner Companies received hundreds of millions of dollars in loans through American companies, including Citigroup and the private equity firm Apollo Global Management, after their top executives met with Kushner in the White House" (Editorial Board, Part 3, 2018). Apollo lent him $134 million, and Citicorp lent $325 million (Drucker, Kelly and Protess, 2018). Prior to these meetings Kushner did not do the due diligence check usual when senior White House officials meet with financial or industrial interests, just as he failed on numerous occasions to fill out security clearance forms completely (Cassidy, March 2018). *The Washington Post* quotes William M. Daley, a former White House chief of staff and Department of Commerce secretary under Democratic presidents: "[Jared Kushner], a family member with no experience at anything other than real estate, no real profile other than a family-run business with a shady past, given incredibly complicated tasks, was a joke.... People elect a president knowing so much about them, good or bad, but no one knows Jared Kushner in the game he is playing. The fact that he made so many blunders, starting with the back-channel talks with Russians, should have told one how in over his head he was" (Rucker, Parker and Dawsey, 2018). At least President John Adams's son had been a diplomat!

Nepotism Continued

It is a quandary whether to include a discussion of Dr. Ben Carson's $31,000 dining room table purchase for his office, purchased by his wife, in this section on Donald Trump's "Nepotism," or reserve it for a section titled, "Bungled and Bumbling Cabinet Appointments." While serving as Housing and Urban Development Secretary, Dr. Carson has invited his investor son, Ben Jr., to HUD meetings that he had no governmental right to attend. In the case of his son, Carson went ahead "over the objections of department lawyers who advised him that the invitation could be seen as a conflict of interest" (Thrush, 2018).

In a hearing before the House Appropriations subcommittee focusing on HUD's budget, Carson offered no adequate explanation as to why his wife was assigned a responsibility easily and ordinarily handled by a government aide, nor justification presented for the outrageous cost. Dr. Carson's several varying and contradictory explanations have been outlined in *The New York Times*, "the committee argued that Mr. Carson's timeline suggested that he was simultaneously outraged by the high cost of the set—and ignorant of the price tag" (Thrush, 2018). Answering criticisms of his son's presence at government meetings, Carson issued this astonishing statement, "HUD's ethics counsel suggested it might look funny, but I'm not a person who spends a lot of time thinking about how something looks." Respectfully, this neurosurgeon requires an ophthalmologic examination because his behavior clearly "looks" like nepotism, definitely entails bungling, and is further fouled by bumbling explanations.

This governmental social fabric of nepotism appears modeled by the president's open indulgences toward his family, an attitude seemingly and sadly for the rest of us, not lost on his appointees.

What Drives Trump's Nepotism?

Pondering the psychology of Trump's nepotism, we can look to his conviction that family loyalty is of prime importance in preserving one's power and safety in the wider world. Donald J. Trump is more provincial in his comforts than many would think—the penchant for McDonald's burgers hints at his tastes—the move from New York to Washington is drastic. Remember, it took Melania Trump six months to move to Washington; her feelings are not alien to her spouse. And further, recall President Trump's older sister, Judge Maryanne Barry, in 2016 dryly noting of her brother, "He's still just a simple boy from Queens! You can quote me on that" (She had refused any other comment for the reporters.) (Schwartzman and Miller, 2016). Imagine President Trump's anxiety if he were to arrive in Washington alone, without his customary tribal family entourage. Additionally, like his father, Fred C. Trump Sr., he aimed to be the business monarch in a family business. One works not only for oneself, but importantly, with and for the next generation. The young Donald Trump knew how deeply happy his father was as they worked together. Anyone can remember the depth of love experienced in making Mom or Dad happy. When Donald Trump's brother, Robert, joined the Trump Organization it was a wonderful day for Donald; he felt his brother had finally "come home." The business is home. Nepotism is a small word, but it covers tangled regions of the psyche.

This business-family identification is psychologically seamless in President Trump's mind, and does not breech ethical boundaries as erected by those not sharing his mind set. What seems incredible to others is totally acceptable to President Trump and no more than "business as usual."

I wonder, however, if President Trump's flourishing under his father's boundless confidence might blind him in relation to his own children. Are they of the same material? The president may—oddly enough, given his ego—underestimate his own rarity, and be misapplying Fred C. Trump Sr.'s correctly applied confidence in the wrong quarters.

Mixing Business with Public Service

The diligence of a major, national accounting firm, additionally aided by in-house lawyers, are required to do adequate justice to the ethical and legal infringements indulged by President Donald J. Trump with his mixture of business and public service. One doesn't need to be a certified public accountant nor be a lawyer, however, to have concerns over several glaring issues.

Despite promises all through his campaign to the contrary, Donald Trump has not issued his personal tax returns; all presidents in the past forty years have done so. What questions does that lack of transparency raise? With what foreign businesses might Trump have financial relationships? And connected with such businesses, what are their inevitable ties to foreign governments? Could these relationships affect his international policies, if not directly, then indirectly, even unwittingly? Is there a Russia connection? Any offshore tax dodges? What are his charitable contributions? Charitable, out of pocket giving, often gives an understanding of personal values. If there is nothing to hide, why is it still hidden? The issue is not idle curiosity; I don't care a bit about how rich Donald Trump is. But I want concrete assurances that Donald J. Trump's conduct as president is not subject to the unavoidable tentacles of a well-established, worldwide business.

The blind trust purportedly set up for the president is not blind; he is free to receive disbursements "on request," as per the few documents available to the public. Therefore, he knows what the profits are, what money he is drawing, and how the business is doing—hardly blind. Plus, his son, Eric (one of the trustees assigned to run Trump Organization), has indicated he talks to his father about how the Trump Organization is doing. Forbes reports that Eric Trump "concedes that he will continue to update his father on the business" while Donald Trump is president. Eric Trump described his reporting to his father, "Yeah, on the bottom line, profitability reports and stuff like that, but you know, that's about it." How often will those reports be every quarter? "Depending.... probably quarterly.... My father and I are very close.... I talk to him a lot. We're pretty inseparable" (Alexander, 2017).

President Trump's disregard of protective ethical standards seems arrogant and intolerant of government standards; ethics protect everyone. We are all human, capable of being influenced, including the president.

It is troubling that practically all of President Donald J. Trump's free time is spent at some Trump branded business, and that includes the club portion of Mar-a-Largo as well as a long string of Trump owned golf clubs. The Trump International Hotel Washington, down the street from the White House, is difficult to mentally digest. The Trump name has ensured a full contingent of foreign envoys, lobbyists, seekers of influence, and an unending bevy of curious tourists, all to the profit of the Trump Organization.

"At the bar of the Trump International Hotel in Washington, you can order a crystal spoonful of Hungarian wine for $140. Cocktails run from $23 for a gin and tonic to $100 for a vodka concoction with raw oysters and caviar. There's a seafood pyramid called 'the Trump Tower' that costs $120, or you can hit BLT Prime, a restaurant where the $59 salt-aged Kansas City strip steak comes with a long-shot chance of seeing the president sitting nearby. It's the only restaurant in town where he has dined. If the urge to shop strikes, there's a Brioni boutique in one corner that offers the same Italian suits the president favors, starting at a few thousand a pop. Downstairs, a 90-minute couple's massage at the spa will set you back $460—roughly the rack rate for a recent night in a standard room, where the Trump brand adorns everything from the shampoo bottles to the wine in the minibar" (Altman, 2017). To avoid overt conflict of interest, the profits from this hotel are poured back into the hotel itself, capital improvements, and profits are not dispensed to the Trump Organization. But, clearly, the value of this property goes up and up, and accrues to the asset wealth of Trump Organization.

The gift of $151,000 in profit from all other Trump hotels and properties from foreign government business, for the full year of 2017, paid to the U.S. Treasury, is accordingly difficult to comprehend—don't they make more money? Perhaps they need new management.

The New York Times reports that during his presidency, one out of three days President Trump has spent at one of his properties, which includes charges by his security personnel to his businesses (for example, $137,000 for their golf carts in one recent three-month period). The club at Mar-a-Lago has doubled its membership fee to $200,000. Plus, "The president personally intervened in a plan to relocate the FBI's Washington headquarters, apparently to protect Trump International Hotel, which is about a block away. If the FBI had moved, its current site would most likely have been turned into a commercial development, and the long construction process—as well as potential for a new hotel on the site—could have hurt the Trump hotel" (Leonhardt and Philbrick, 2018).

What can one make of such egregious disregard of time-tested governmental rules of conduct and ethical guidelines? What might be President Trump's psychological perspective that supports this disregard of historical caution and ring of safeguards slowly accumulated through national experience? I can only imagine that President Trump acts out of a lifetime of jungle business experience in New York and international business. In those settings, although setbacks and failures were aplenty, on the whole, to President Trump, his upward trajectory reads: self-directed, counter-expected-behaviors lead to success despite predicted failure by "experts." He lurches forward bulwarked by an inner aggressiveness well rationalized through long, intimate experience with his father's business tactics, reinforced with a moral fortitude supplied by Reverend Peale (Trump has the assurance of a man buoyed by faith-based precepts), and years of crafty reliance on wily legal maps charting judicial routes avoided by most citizens.

I do not believe President Trump sees himself as engaging in anything deleterious to the nation, certainly nothing remotely criminal, but believes his uncanny understanding and management of events will result in the betterment of all Americans. If his business and those associated with his family prosper, that is not a motive of any consequence to him, it is merely incidental. In President Trump's mind, all these transgressions, important to others, are irrelevant motes of oppositional detail compared to his succeeding vision of a rescued American. The ship of state will rise. In a strange irony, he anticipates a flourishing of the maxim of a Democratic Party icon, President John F. Kennedy: "A rising tide lifts all the boats."

Immigration and Immigrants

Ripping apart several million families runs the risk of repeating the tragedies of slavery from which our nation has still not recovered. Many illegal aliens have children who are American citizens by birth and thus are entitled to all American rights and privileges. The parents and much of their extended family do not.

Deportation of these parents and other close relatives and friends of the children thus leading to traumatic fracturing of families and communities is a recipe for national psychological disaster. We must learn from the tragic history of African-American slavery where such family and social dissolution was commonplace.

I concur with President Trump that illegal aliens with criminal records should be deported, but they are a small fraction of the nation's eleven million illegal immigrants. The vast majority of illegals are not criminal, and labeling them as such is equivalent to declaring them guilty until proven innocent. If one has any inclination toward assimilating aliens into our nation, beginning with an abrogation of American civil liberties is a grim introduction to our way of life.

I support carefully planned and detailed schedules toward citizenship for all illegal aliens already present in our country. The end goal would be for all illegal aliens to become citizens within a specific time frame, somewhere between three and five years. There could be room for speedier pathways for those who have done military service or other equivalent laudatory public service. Or, all illegal aliens who haven't done prior, adequate public service, might be required to offer unpaid community service while they are preparing for citizenship, perhaps two years, like military duty. If they do not complete the program and become naturalized citizens, then they are deported. And, I am for instituting monetary fines for the crime of illegal entry, payable over time, perhaps, but citizenship is not granted without payment. I am proposing a financial penalty payment as well as restitute community service for two years. The goal of these programs is assimilation, to bring people of merit out of the shadows and allowed their full potential to contribute to America.

As part of the process outlined, a revamped, vigorous immigration policy, including stricter border controls, would be designed to close the door on further, nation straining, illegal immigration.

Inept Appointments and Non-Appointments

There is no way to countenance the appointment of Betsy DeVos as Secretary of Education. Since Donald Trump ran a campaign as defender of the defenseless, a voice for the working poor, how could he believe a person who was destroying public education could meet their needs? As repeatedly demonstrated, embarrassingly and painfully, in Congressional hearings, Ms. DeVos has little knowledge of educational facts and statistics. Apart from diverting departmental energies and personnel from investigating fraudulent "for profit" educational institutions, which she has formerly championed and invested in, she has been fostering policies that block their former "scammed" students from forgiveness for their educational loans. There are now 100,000 such cases outstanding. Perhaps it is not just incidental that, in the past, DeVos has also invested financially in student-loan-debt-collection businesses (Cowley, 2018).

Equally distressing is the appointment of Dr. Ben Carson as Secretary to Housing and Urban Development (HUD). I have already cited Dr. Carson's errant nepotism as a quandary as a public servant, but one of our greatest American crises is homelessness, along with decreased affordable housing, and frightening urban decay. For such an awesome, national, social epidemic, increasing in degree, how can Dr. Carson, who has spent his life in cloistered, windowless, operating rooms, be versed in HUD's urban challenges (Salzillio, 2017) (Shapiro, 2018)? While President Trump is perhaps paying back campaign chits to Dr. Carson, President Trump is blindly robbing his most defenseless and poorest citizens of skilled, well-informed, experienced help. "[HUD is] scaling back federal efforts to enforce fair housing laws, freezing enforcement actions against local governments and businesses...while sidelining officials who have aggressively pursued civil rights cases" (Thrush, 2018).

Fortunately, unrelenting light focused on the shadowy activities of Secretary of the Interior Ryan Zinke and he is now gone. The inspector general of the Interior found several issues concerning Zinke warranted referral to the Department of Justice for criminal investigation. Briefly, *The New York Times* detailed activities of Secretary Zinke and his wife concerning land deals, particularly in Montana, that suggest they used their power at the Interior to enrich themselves (Eilperin, Dawsey and Rein, 2018). Although Trump may have been quietly satisfied that Zinke was pursing Trump's agenda with coal, oil, and gas production, apparently Zinke pushed the ethical envelope too far.

Although Scott Pruitt resigned from his post as Secretary of the Environmental Protection Agency in July 2018, he left behind a troubling cloud of questions. His alleged transgressions include a potpourri of charges concerning lavish spending for travel and purchases, questionable relationships with lobbyists, possible use of his office to influence business opportunities for his wife, and staff turmoil (about a dozen people resigned). For a long while as Secretary of the EPA he vigorously pursued a policy of deregulation that was proving to be the largest in his agency's history. This pursuit of policies favored by Trump was not enough to hold the president's support as scandal after scandal mounted. Toward the end of his tenure there were reports of Pruitt angling for the job of Attorney General (prior to the resignation of Jeff Sessions). Perhaps it was this latter issue that became the straw that broke the political camel's back for President Trump who finally let him go (Davenport, Friedman and Haberman, 2018).

There is no shortage of other violations of public trust by appointed members of the administration, some accompanied by well-deserved resignations, but I will stop with the foregoing as the point is clear. President Trump's self-confidence about spotting appropriate, talented people based on his years of business experience has not quite carried over into Washington. I can foresee a complication to learning on-the-job about the abilities and disabilities of the governmental, and that is President Trump's stubbornness and anxiety about not following his "proven" playbook. This "playbook" includes cutting your losses with an abrupt firing. Psychologically, Trump is not a good candidate for turnaround thinking in assessing candidates for office, although this same ease of change is a remarkable asset in negotiations. It could take Trump the rest of his term in office to slowly, incrementally, become familiar with the political landscape and recognize good candidates for office. Whether this handicap will suffice to block his overall vision for America is a question that has yet to be answered.

Hobbling the State Department

In a world of increasing size of great nations (China, India), and due to local nationalism, a simultaneous rise in the number of small nations (see the UN roster), it makes little sense to leave so many posts, major and minor, vacant in our State Department. As of February 2018, thirteen months into the presidency, fifty-seven ambassadorial posts remained vacant (Sit, 2018). In June 2018, 500 days into the Trump presidency, more than forty top jobs in the state department still remained unfilled. Dozens of Obama ambassadorial appointees were fired by Trump when he took office and few replaced (Schoen, 2018). The delays in appointments are longer than the previous past six administrations. Although President Trump began surprise negotiations with North Korea, we, amazingly, still did not have a permanent Ambassador to South Korea until June 30, 2018. Continuing to enjoy his trust in the military, President Trump chose retired U.S. Navy Admiral Harry B. Harris, former commander of the U.S. Pacific Command. Ambassador Harris has the official title of Ambassador Extraordinary and Plenipotentiary of the United States of America to the Republic of Korea.

I cannot reconcile this State Department decay with President Trump's electioneering promises of decreasing governmental bureaucracy. Diplomatic relationships do not turn on a dime. Delaying this process of diplomatic acculturation keeps us in the dark about foreign issues and cripples informed planning concerning foreign matters that have an impact on our nation. President Trump's brand of uncompromising international isolationism may be sowing the seeds of calamitous global diplomatic disadvantages.

It is quite possible that Trump's long and successful business experience with personal control over every detail has misled him into thinking the same hold true in government. Giving up control and delegating authority in the State Department is particularly foggy for President Trump. Judgment concerning nominees depends on knowledge of lands and people totally foreign to the president. President Trump depends on loyalty, and how can one judge loyalty in this unusual group of people, many of whom, the most qualified, have spent their time and their relationships far, far from home? Loyalty requires the test of time, and state department appointments will flow in proportion to Trump's comfort with the nominees, their loyalty, which comes only painstakingly through time.

LGBTQ – Gun Control

LGBTQ rights and Gun Control are two topics of great concern and have been treated poorly by President Trump and his administration. I feel, however, that both issues have been caught in the crossfire of electioneering politics due to the Republican Party's anxiety over mid-term elections of 2018, and I fear that Republican losses after the November 2018 election will lead to more stagnating, inter-political-party fruitless wrangling on both these issues. I group these issues together not because they are similar at all, but each bears a unique vulnerability to political haggling and deal making. They have been each sacrificed by the Trump administration for political gains. Each issue is complex, with wide social and psychological ramifications, involves passionately held opinions and not uncommonly includes violent feelings. A properly respectful presentation of these matters is not possible in a brief overview.

I must acknowledge, however, that before the presidency, Trump's life reflected open support of the LGBTQ community. In 2016, "candidate Trump presented himself as a social liberal seeking to move the Republican Party left on gay, lesbian, bisexual, and transgender rights. He vowed that he would do more than Democrat Hillary Clinton to protect LGBT people. He defended the rights of Caitlyn Jenner, the country's most well-known transgender advocate, to use whichever bathroom she wanted in Trump Tower. And he added "Q" to his discussion of the 'LGBTQ community' in his Republican National Convention speech to show he was in the know" (Samuels and Johnson, 2017). One prominent gay leader, Gregory T. Angelo of the Log Cabin Republicans had labeled candidate Trump the "most pro-LGBT Republican nominee in history," but noted that LGBTQ rights had fallen victim to "politics" in the Trump administration.

We have seen that in Trump's personal history, he had no difficulty trusting Roy Cohn with the most intimate details and secrets of his financial and romantic life. Early in their intense relationship Trump understood that Cohn was a "closeted" gay—and this unconflicted acceptance was long before it was fashionable or politically correct. Further, gays have held and hold executive positions in Trump Organization. The Mar-a-Largo Club, against much local opposition, was the first Palm Beach country club publicly open to gays, lesbians, as well as

African Americans. Mar-a-Lago was also first in accepting gay couples. Nowhere in Donald Trump's life was gay or lesbian a troubling issue for him.

And with gun control, President Trump's February 2018's startling proposal of comprehensive gun control measures—promulgated on live TV and with Diane Feinstein sitting next to him, smiling—were backed down from in the face of stiff political opposition, primarily from his Republican colleagues (Shear, 2018). Since then, President Trump has leaned back into a stance fully supported by the National Rifle Association. Given the unending gun tragedies that agonize all levels of our society, a serious grappling of the problem by Congress is very long overdue and quite negligent of public safety. I await President Trump's return to his startling February 2018 proposals. I am assuming we are in the early innings of an unseen process of political bargaining, and at a more propitious time, we will see a return of his active engagement for the necessary progressive measures for the LGBTQ community and gun control. It is possible Trump may require re-election in 2020 to garner sufficient political power to effect significant change on either issue. Ironically, newly found Democratic leverage may provide him an unexpected liberal pathway before then. Democrats may find Trump uncannily (and politically wily) receptive on these issues.

Outrageous Behavior

America now knows how Fred Trump Sr. felt when, after years of hearing school complaints about his son, Donald's, incorrigible behavior, he finally capitulated and sent Donald to a military school. Where do we send the president of the United States? West Point? Too old. Guantanamo? He would drive the guards insane with tweets.

Optimistic pundits hoped that the gravitas of the presidential office would mellow, mold, and mature his impulsive antics (just like his father held similar hopes about military school). There was no such luck. These behaviors have been locked in since early childhood. Trump labeled his unrelenting childhood antics as "aggressive" and clearly this openly hard-hitting proclivity never abated. The locus of the outrageous conduct may have changed from Trump Tower to the White House, but not the focus: disloyalty and opposition.

Trump's style of handling dissent during his business years included not only schemes to vanquish his opponent, but, often included revenge. This almost axiomatic destructive counter-coup was most evident when a close business associate engaged in disloyal behavior. Objection to Jeff Sessions's recusal from the Mueller investigation of Russian collusion centered on a loyalty issue. Trump was outraged that Sessions did not see that his first order of business as Attorney General of the United States was loyalty to the president. The two were barely on speaking terms for most of Sessions's tenure as Attorney General. Loyalty to America was missing. When Secretary of State Rex Tillerson disagreed with President Trump on several diplomatic fronts it was not only opposition, but a multitude of antitheses that amounted to open disloyalty.

Once Trump has deemed someone "disloyal," the person is never trusted again. Disloyalty is worse than opposition. During the primaries and presidential election, Ted Cruz was an opponent. But during the 2018 midterms Trump unabashedly and enthusiastically campaigned for him. Disloyalty is a loss of power, whereas opposition is fickle.

President Trump's negotiating depends on an "anchoring bias"—starting from an extreme position and compromising downward. Thus, his initial approach with Kim Jong-un had the extreme stance of "no negotiation with a terrorist nation," and no shortage of ridicule of "Little Rocket Man." In Trump's mind, he's in control of the negotiation. When North Korea shifted its stance and seemed more diplomatically accessible, Trump easily backed off from threats of war, offered negotiations, and even threw in declarations of "love" for Kim Jong-un.

Trump also faces many issues essentially beyond his control. On these relatively uncontrollable matters he can take an extreme, irrational view and hold it, even if through the years he may have expressed the opposite view. Political catering to his conservative base is his strategic choice. We saw this surprising reversal with gun control, formerly more liberal (or left, depending on your viewpoint) and also with LGBTQ. This need to hold a blatant political view creates bizarre, unpalatable platforms like the one suggesting there is only a binary reality to gender, a person is always only one of two genders at birth. This is patent medical nonsense; for example, what about persons born with intersex characteristics?

Distortion, denial, and blaming from politicians may be distressing, disheartening, and depressing, but in small doses the voters digest and forget over time. But, unfortunately, President Trump continually floods us with incredible, outlandish, unproved claims—a sampling includes bused-in illegal out-of-state voters, record tax changes; seventeen people conducting the Mueller investigation worked in Hillary Clinton connected ventures; the governments of Guatemala and Honduras were complicit in forming caravans of migrants (plus a host of distortions used to support his disastrous, humanly cruel, government shutdown of 2018–2019); a bizarre blaming of California for mismanagement of forests to explain its tragic fires when, in fact, the federal government owns 75 percent of the California forests; and, so on. The list is long, troubling, and shows no signs of abating.

I am far from a fan of the negative editorial policy of *The Washington Post* in regard to President Trump, but I quote the following since it captures my distress:

> *On Sept. 7, 2018 President Trump woke up in Billings, Mont., flew to Fargo, N.D., visited Sioux Falls, S.D., and eventually returned to Washington. He spoke to reporters on Air Force One, held a pair of fundraisers and was interviewed by three local reporters. In that single day, he publicly made 125 false or misleading statements—in a period of time that totaled only about 120 minutes. It was a new single-day high. The day before, the president made 74 false or misleading claims… Trump's tsunami of untruths helped push the count in The Fact Checker's database past 5,000 on the 601st day of his presidency. That's an average of 8.3 Trumpian claims a day, but in the past nine*

> *days—the president has averaged 32 claims a day (Kessler, Rizzo and Kelly, 2018).*

How to tolerate such insupportable conduct? In truth, it is always painful. I can only speculate that Trump's consistent outbursts of linguistic aggression helps maintain his mental balance by affording him the feelings of a victor on his way to victory while believing his claims are shared by ardent followers; the solitary tweeter has a multitude of supporters. If this letting off of aggressive steam and soothing distortion of facts allows President Trump the necessary mental balance to achieve greater goals for the nation, then historically it will be blended into the national benefits received. If not, this conduct is totally unredeemable and will remain a blemish on our national standards of conduct. And, even if it is redeemed, in my lifetime at least, it will continue to feel outrageous.

Misgivings Versus Misguided

This book has tried to marshal positive and reassuring features of President Donald Trump's life and personality. These features can offer assurance that President Trump is psychologically sound, capable, competent, and dedicated to strengthening our nation. As good as he is, however, he is like the rest of us, human. He is subject to his own shortcomings, be they experiential or biologically constitutional, plus he is subject to the shortcomings of our cantankerous government. One may have a horrific opinion of American government, but keep in mind Winston Churchill's observation: "Democracy is the worst form of Government except for all those other forms that have been tried from time to time."

It is important to be aware of differences with someone we support. In Trump's case, the differences clarify issues I support and those I don't. Support is not a blanket endorsement. I am not expecting President Trump to see all sides of an issue, or to always be able to maneuver politically on all issues. It is part of my role as a responsible citizen to recognize my differences, and make them known if I have any hope of having them carry weight. In effect, differences can enhance realistic support rather than blind adherence. Articulated differences, communicated differences, will inform and influence elected officials, including the president. The ballot box needs support both before and after pulling the lever.

CHAPTER

8

INSUFFICIENT AWE

Awe

Awe connotes a mysterious mixture of comprehension and incomprehension, reverence, respect, wonder, astonishment, and on its edges, fear. Whether we were a small rag-tag band of battling ex-colonists or a present-day burgeoning world power of over 330 million people, our national psychology seeks a supreme leader—albeit modulated by the checks and balances outlined by our founders. The presidential mantle in and of itself evokes awe.

If we add to this mantle the unexpected fringe of an outsider victor, the awe becomes one unique to President Donald Trump. Never having held any public office in the first seventy years of his life, he now holds the one most revered and desired.

JP Morgan CEO Jaime Dimon was considered for Secretary of the Treasury in Trump's administration, but declined interest. In September 2016 Dimon was asked if he would like to be president of the United States, replying "Yeah, I would have.... But the time has passed. I always thought you had to have government experience, be a state governor or a senator, and I never had that.... But then I look at Donald J. Trump [who won the Republican nomination], and I think, 'See! What do I know!'" (Isidore, 2016).

The Outsider

It is a special quality of Donald Trump's character to be most comfortable as an outsider. His life history contains an extensive list of winning long shot business opportunities. As he struck out on his own, beyond the established safety of his father Fred's Queens/Brooklyn business, that a young Donald knew well, and chose to venture over the East River into Manhattan, his father strongly urged him not to try his luck in what Fred Sr. considered an overpriced and excessively risky real estate market. Ever self-confident, Trump began in Manhattan as a one-man operation. Early major real estate ventures were battles against lack of personal recognition (the Hyatt hotel, Trump Tower, 40 Wall Street, the West Side residential development). He fought New York City politicians and Mayor Ed Koch even for charitable offerings (Wollman Skating Rink). Later, many associates strongly advised against his involvement in what was then a new TV production, *The Apprentice*. Colleagues predicted failure in a television role for which he lacked experience and knowledge. Over fourteen highly successful seasons of *The Apprentice*, Donald Trump earned $214 million, and in the process also contributed a now well-known phrase to the American linguistic lexicon: "You're fired!" Interestingly, in that TV program's scenario he recreated a central piece of his own experience and central identity: Only one person, an unknown, against difficult odds, became the winner.

Some outsider positions did end in drastic failure (such as his Atlantic City casinos), but he remained undaunted, and continued building, creating the *TRUMP* brand. Trump forged ahead in his campaign for the presidency, girded with first-hand experience as an outsider and familiarity with frustration linked to his continuous drive for success as an unproven, unknown interloper. This outsider characteristic gave Trump a natural and intuitive empathy with voters who felt unrecognized, unheard, and cut off from political power. A social psychological resonance of campaigner with voters was natural, unforced, intuitive, and genuine. Trump knew one could come from behind and win; he convincingly conveyed the same to his voters. He meant it when he implored that they and he could, "Make America Great Again."

Trump's Appeal

In an unusual combination—awesome in its uniqueness—Donald Trump appealed to the working class, wealthy conservatives, and the battle-hardened military. Once again, I emphasize that Trump spent most of his first twenty-seven years of life in Queens and Brooklyn, in close contact with carpenters, plumbers, electricians, plasterers, stone masons, painters, bricklayers, roofers, glaziers, truckers, and so on. He understands everyday work life, everyday frustrations, and especially, everyday speech. His wealthy persona is more familiar to people, especially through the fourteen years of his highly successful and widely viewed show, *The Apprentice*. One must also not underestimate the impact of spending formative adolescent years in military school. It was not combat, but it was the world of the military, and he shone in it, garnering respect and awards. Belief in the necessity of the military has a long, personal history with Trump, and his support is conveyed with conviction to our military and veterans.

The outsider position fits with Trump's need for privacy and the use of the persona as a socially protective shield. They are two unchangeable sides of Trump. Combining both these traits effectively has allowed Trump to attain great power and great wealth, achievements that add to his awe. This psychological safety of being the solitary outsider trusting long odds playing out in his favor, while simultaneously representing the burgeoning needs of a large group (Trump Organization now numbers over 20,000 people) has carried into his management of the role of president faced with the needs of the nation. For Trump, the past dictates the present.

It is a sad irony of the psychology of the outsider that no matter how much they achieve entry to a fantasied insider status they still lovingly hold onto the special independent nature of their different roots as a basic identity. Trump's older sister, Maryanne, shared the essence of her understanding of her brother in 2016, "He's still just a simple boy from Queens. You can quote me on that." The Reverend Al Sharpton knew Trump well from the New York years also epitomized Trump as an "outsider" from Queens seeking a place among the elite, and never fully feeling it even after building Trump Tower (Kranish, 2019). And quite tellingly, in the recent *New York Times* interview between its publisher A. G. Sulzberger and Trump, near the end of the interview, Trump lamented to Sulzberger that although "I come from New York...I love New York...I started from Queens," yet, a favorite (perhaps former favorite) hometown newspaper had failed to write a story he deeply desired: How a local boy from Jamaica Estates, Queens had become president of the United States (Grynbaum, 2019).

Fear of the Outsider

While outsider status appeals to democratic longings for eventual inclusion to the "inner circle," it also invokes fear of the unknown, the unproven, and the unpredictable. Wealth and power, especially to those without it, adds to the mystery of awe. In this emotional cloud, keeping campaign promises is paramount to stem fear among Trump supporters, and to his credit, despite many obstacles, President Trump tries to redeem campaign promises. For example, rescinding the Iran nuclear pact combines many of his campaign pledges, including separating us from the leverage of European diplomacy. A long desired Republican tax reform plan was delivered, and it's ultimate goal of increasing general prosperity is yet to be fully demonstrated. Similarly, immigration reform—including "the wall"—satisfying humanistic principles, and yet not sacrificing national identity and law, remains an unfinished challenge, but is never absent from Trump's active efforts.

A major threat to our government has been the unfettered growth of federal bureaucracy, the so-called "fourth branch" of government. Unelected bureaucrats have attained quasi-legislative powers as they interpret gray areas of regulatory control. This administrative state has become an ever-expanding fourth branch of government in a de facto fashion never imagined by our founding fathers. In a 2016 summary of this burgeoning problem, some examples were "the IRS (which is responsible for the ridiculous 70,000-page tax code that has crippled small businesses)...to the Environmental Protection Agency (which has instituted over 3,000 pages of federal regulations on energy output that has decimated the energy market) to the Department of Veterans Affairs (which is responsible for extraordinarily backlogging disability appeals, denying mental health services to over 125,000 veterans, and extending the wait-list for first time applicants to three years and over)" (Vasquez, 2016). In an editorial, the *Washington Examiner* decried the rising practice of Environmental Protection Agency scientists, lawyers, and experts banding together like lobbyists to influence senators in their choice of nominations to head the agency (Editorial Board, 2017).

President Trump has effectively supported decreased regulation, and importantly, appointed, and continues to appoint, federal judges and supreme court justices who will support further deregulation. This stance ultimately restores encroached freedoms to citizens. The impact of this judicial change will be powerful, and Trump's judicial legacy will be evident for at least a generation, beyond his presidency, whether he is re-elected in 2020 or not.

Isolationism and American Survival

President Trump's overarching principle is "America First." This principle is behind the economic saber rattling of tariffs, reducing America's military activities as the world's police force and proselytizer of American-style democracy, a reduction in funding to the United Nations and NATO, separating us from the international diplomacy of Europe, tightening immigration policies, and becoming energy independent. The enormity of this change in American internationalism was suggested by former Secretary of State Henry Kissinger when he commented that "I think Trump may be one of those figures in history who appears from time to time to mark the end of an era and to force it to give up its old pretenses. It doesn't necessarily mean that he knows this, or that he is considering any great alternative. It could just be an accident" (Luce, 2018). Kissinger's deep perspective is highlighted in a new book by Hanson, *The Case for Trump* (2019). Hanson elaborates how "Trump [has] the instincts and energy… to dismantle…and bring long-overdue policy changes at home and abroad. We could not survive a series of presidencies as volatile as Trump's. But after decades of drift, America needs the outsider Trump to do what usual politicians would not or could not do" (King, 2019). A historic momentum may be catapulting us all toward change, but it is President Trump who embodies its goals and uniquely has his hands on the baton of change.

Mirroring President Trump's emphasis on protective nationalism versus assertive internationalism is the recent unusual appearance of three books echoing cautious halting of liberal globalism: John Mearsheimer, *The Great Delusion: Liberal Dreams and International Realities*; Jeffrey Sachs, *A New Foreign Policy: Beyond American Exceptionalism;* Stephen Walt, *The Hell of Good Intentions: America's Foreign Policy Elite and the Decline of US Primacy*.

In summarizing their content, *The Boston Globe* review stated, "In their new books, all three of these heretics pronounce American foreign policy a failure. They assert that the drive for 'full-spectrum dominance,' on which we have been embarked since the Cold War ended a quarter-century ago, has destabilized the world and undermined our own security.... Stephen Walt, the dissenting realist at Harvard's John F. Kennedy School of Government, [believes] pursuing liberal hegemony [assertive actions in the world to implant American democracy, free markets, and human rights] did not make the United States safer, stronger, more prosperous, or more popular.... On the contrary, America's ambitious attempt to reorder world politics undermined its own position, sowed chaos in several regions, and caused considerable misery in a number of other countries.... Mearsheimer...tells us that people everywhere are moved more by nationalism than liberal idealism.... American politicians should remind voters that, since nationalism places great emphasis on self-determination, patriots in other countries will inevitably rebel if we try to dominate them.... Liberal hegemony does not satisfy the principal criterion for assessing any foreign policy: it is not in America's national interest.... Walt marvels that government officials and commentators who promote disastrous wars not only suffer no consequences, but are welcomed back into circles of power—it is the dissidents and critics who end up marginalized or penalized, even when they are proved right" (Kinzer, 2018). Sound familiar? President Trump is constantly under threat of penalization (the craze for impeachment is the ultimate form) and efforts to marginalize him have been made by both Republicans and Democrats. The psychology of the repulsed "outsider" is painful, particularly in Trump who craves adulation, but it provides unshakeable confidence—he has been down this road many times before and come out on top.

In an era when globalism is promoted as social progress, President Trump's nationalism will be cardinal to the continued growth, development, and survival of America. The great empires of the past, the Roman, the Spanish, and the English, all came to be economically dependent on distant lands, lands that were ultimately lost, and with that loss, their source of greatness. Trump's policies with an emphasis on independence will protect America from the often-predicted doomed fate of earlier "great" empires.

Western Europe's Immigration Crisis

The calamitous civil plight of many Western European countries overwhelmed by Muslim immigration has neither excited nor attracted media attention in the United States. The terrible suffering of the immigrants at the United States southwestern border has dominated reporting. To a large extent, the physical barriers provided by several thousands of miles of oceans on either side of our geography has helped ward off the same kind of invasion that Europe has seen. Americans have not directly felt the pain of the frightening events in Europe, and consequently America remains in an uninformed bubble reminiscent of the safely buffered, unknowing climate in the years prior to World War II.

In western European countries such as Germany, France, Belgium, the Scandinavian nations, especially Sweden, there are increasing episodes of jihadist and other forms of violence. Countries with tighter immigration controls, such as Poland, the Czech Republic, Hungary, and Austria have all been spared the carnage. There are also issues resulting from the cultural clash between Islam and the West. Few Westerners are comfortable with importing polygamy, childhood marriages, misogyny, female genital mutilation, the grooming of adolescents for sex trafficking, and Sharia Law (Bennhold, June 2018) (Cat, 2018) (Geller, August 6, 2018) (Geller, August 14, 2018) (Geller, August 16, 2018) (Geller, August 19, 2018) (Geller, August 24, 2018) (Kern, June 2018) (Kern, July 2018) (Kern, August 2018) (Meotti, April 2018) (Voice of Europe, June 2018).

Muslim neighborhoods known as "no-go zones" have developed where police or civil agencies like fire departments will not enter, fearful of mob attacks. In such "no-go zones" there is wholesale rejection of Western European law, government, and culture. The government of France has finally admitted the existence of 1,500 such "sensitive urban zones" and estimates a population within them of six million—roughly one-tenth of France (Kern, November 2017) (King, 2018) (Meotti, August 2018) (Voice of Europe, June 2018) (Voice of Europe, July 2018).

Concomitant with these anti-Western actions is a frightening rise of anti-Semitism causing an escalating flight of Jews from western Europe. Once again, fleeing Jews may be the cultural canaries in the international coalmine (Boyes, 2017) (Hurd, 2015) (Pour, 2018) (Smith-Spark, 2018).

In 2004, one of the Western world's foremost Islamic scholars, Bernard Lewis, presciently, and for those naïve times, shockingly, offered the German newspaper *Die Welt* the opinion, "Europe will be Islamic by the end of the century" (McCarthy, 2017). Close on Lewis's scholarly heels, in 2006, from a somewhat equally informed Islamic source were the words of the late Libyan autocrat, Muammar Gaddafi, "We have fifty million Muslims in Europe. There are signs [of an] Islam victory in Europe—without swords, without guns, without conquests. The fifty millions of Europe will turn it into a Muslim continent within a few decades" (Gaddafi, 2006) (Kern, December 2017). Militant as he was, even Gaddafi could not envision the recent massive migration and its embedded eruption of jihadi terrorism—complete with all manner of swords, guns, and explosives.

The political split between Western Europe and Eastern Europe—represented by the rise of anti-immigration right-wing parties in Austria, Poland, Czech Republic, and Hungary—possibly presages the outburst of open civil wars within the individual nations of Western Europe. Increasingly, right-wing political strength and challenge, often physically violent, is taking hold in western European countries. Even Chancellor Angela Merkel, the foremost architect of Germany's Syrian refugee program who virtually ignored her country's "no-go zones," finally conceded that they exist, but did so only when her political power was threatened by right-wing opposition election successes. Merkel's utopian dream of invigorating assimilation may be veering toward a nightmare of violence that could embroil much of Western Europe (Bennhold and Eddy, 2018) (Bennhold, August 2018) (Duke, 2018) (Kern, September 2018).

In a fascinating testimony to the central importance of boundaries in national and international politics, President James K. Polk and President Donald J. Trump arrived at similar crossroads. Polk was reviled as he extended our boundaries and Trump is reviled as he seeks to protect them. Both these chief executives fought congressional opposition over boundaries and their management as essential to national interests, power, and safety. In time, if Europe erupts in civil violence, president Trump's seemingly "un-Liberal" protective policies will be viewed as sparing the United States a similar fate.

My prior recommendations for granting citizenship to current illegal immigrants—who are rather assimilated, does not contradict or counter these concerns of the jihadist threat. The issue is not an anti-immigration policy as such—our nation thrives and survives on the imaginative energies of immigrants whatever their culture or religion. I believe immigration is an essential ingredient in the best American virtues. Muslims enrich America in unique ways as does every other immigrant group. Rather, the issue is one of optimal assimilation. Immigration policy and law needs to respect the social psychological capacities of our nation, and Trump's views lean in that direction.

The Overhang of Business

Although Trump's experience in business is often downgraded as a useful model for national government, his path in politics reflects his business style. The Trump Organization never took in partners; it was basically a one-man show, independent. In later years the Trump Organization even eschewed the use of bank financing, funding projects out of its own cash flow, reversing a pattern of incurring debt through his long real estate career. In the nine years prior to his presidential campaign Trump Organization used $400 million of its own money for fourteen different projects. His son, Eric, has suggested that his father's earlier painful, bruising bank debt influenced the change (O'Connell, Farenthold and Gillum, 2018). While increasing national debt flies in the face of this last proposition—for example, increasing the mushrooming military budget—the innate message is one of providing protection of international independence. The need for independence is part of Trump's nature, part of his success—as described earlier, his private self—in this instance, personal psychology promotes political policy.

Meet the Press

Who could predict that a campaigner for president, and then a victorious president, could sideline the media, both national and international, and still be viable? Trump, a real estate billionaire in his seventies, has the communication instincts of a millennial. With flair and frequency, he tweets to the American public daily, nightly, and directly. His uncanny use of the internet rivals FDR's introduction of radio fireside chats and JFK's deft use of television. No one recommended this approach; it seems to have come out of nowhere. Again, against all advice from his own staff, against media ridicule and disparagement, he has continued to have a powerful impact with his dedicated audience. Ironically, journalists, the target of Trump's derision, start their day by imbibing and transmitting his early tweeted words. Nightly tweets are transformed into morning headlines. And, I do mean headlines, not brief mentions on page nine of the local paper, or a brief comment by a television news anchor. From the start of his campaign to today, Trump, by himself, elicits a never-ending barrage of media coverage that for others usually requires a small army of marketing professionals. A one-man internet publishing empire at his fingertips, Citizen Trump has bested Citizen Kane at a fraction of the cost. For well over 150 years, campaigners and presidents traveled on railroad trains crisscrossing towns and hamlets to deliver their message eye-to-eye with citizens from the back of the last train car. That form of immediacy has been translated into 280 characters, a political punch line delivered daily. Someone who never held public office has turned the stereotypical long-winded politician's speech on its head.

The deftness with boiling an issue down to 280 characters reminds me of an anecdote that also characterizes Trump's cognitive style. One of his business executives returned from a trip to another city where he had researched a possible real estate investment for the Trump Organization. He sat in Trump's New York Trump Tower office and launched a long, dutiful, detailed report—all the whys and wherefores. After about twenty minutes Trump interrupted him and said, "Just give it to me in 10 words!" The executive replied, "It stinks!"

North Korea, The Middle East, and China

How can it be that the same president who has borne frenzied cries of "Impeach him!" is the same president lauded as a candidate for the Nobel Peace Prize? It is not only Republicans in Congress who have raised the lofty prospect of a medal for President Trump; similar sentiments floated ashore from foreign soil. British Foreign Secretary Brian Johnson raised the prospect, as did the president of South Korea, Moon Jae-in, who insisted that the central actor in the awesome and historic turnaround of events with North Korea's Kim Jong-un was President Trump. Moon Jae-in unequivocally announced, "President Trump should win the Nobel Peace Prize. The only thing we need is peace" (Noack, 2018).

One can debate the course of events that brings us to this transformational opportunity, whether it was eventual economic exhaustion of North Korea or Trump's brinksmanship. The fact remains that Trump is in the diplomatic catbird seat. He has a chance to make the most of an unexpected opportunity. With North Korea's nuclear testing hovering above their heads and near their coasts, South Korea and Japan had begun to live in constant fear prior to Trump's intervention.

The same president whose major political thrust is isolationist is the same president who may bring peace to a large portion of Asia.

A similar unexpected peaceful compromise may be in process in Afghanistan. Over a decade of diplomatic and military efforts had failed to move the Taliban to agree to peace negotiations. As of late January 2019, this agreement may be forthcoming. President Trump took a great risk in promising withdrawal of American forces from Afghanistan to the Taliban, but it has provided peace negotiations never possible in the past. President Trump daringly underwrote the prison release in Pakistan of a revered founder of the Taliban, Mullah Abdul Ghani Baradar, thus giving the Taliban a powerful, trusted presence in the peace talks in Qatar. As with North Korea, only time will tell, but the shift in diplomatic positive possibilities in Afghanistan is equally unexpected and hopeful. Even the ever-Trump-doubting *The New York Times* penned an editorial "End the War in Afghanistan: It is Time to Bring American Soldiers Back Home" (Editorial Board, 2019). Emphasizing the hopeless stagnation, the editorial outlined the staggering numbers of deaths, injuries, human displacements, and destruction over seventeen years of armed conflict as well as close to $6 trillion spent in the war on terrorism. "When Donald Trump ran for the White House, one of his central promises was to rein in overseas military adventurism and focus the country's limited resources on its core strategic priorities.... He is right...to want to scale back a global conflict [the war on terrorism] that appears to have no outer bound.... It is time to face the cruel truth that at best, the war is deadlocked, and at worst, it is hopeless.... The failure of American leaders—civilians and generals through three administrations, from the Pentagon to the State Department to Congress and the White House—to develop and pursue a strategy to end the war ought to be studied for generations. Likewise, all Americans—the news media included—need to be prepared to examine the national credulity or passivity that's led to the longest conflict in modern American history." The boldness of this *New York Times* editorial matches the brave boldness of President Trump, against strong opposition, in facing the tragic consequences of American international militarism.

Nixon's historic opening of doors to China is contrasted with Trump's dramatic closing of doors or fashioning new ones as China seeks world dominance through economic hegemony. Embedded in our battle over trade tariffs is a full-fledged "technological cold war" with China. The entire national and international tech ecosystem is at risk, and concerns go beyond the unfair economics of Chinese subsidies to technological companies and theft of intellectual properties to military and security issues. In a review of this crisis, *Barron's* magazine warns: "The perception is that too much of the information-and-communication-technology supply chain is centered on China. If we are in a conflict and using infrastructure built by China, they could theoretically hit a button and shut off everything. After thirty years of saying companies should optimize supply chains and move some abroad, now we are saying it's a security concern. Adjusting to that is jarring" (Kapadia, 2019). The champion on the world scene for this confrontation is President Trump whose strength of resolve toward China's policies uniquely challenges the acquiescing accommodations of other major nations.

Throughout all of President Trump's presidential campaign the cry of his international ignorance was raised endlessly. Against the odds, Trump's unexpected challenge of China, sidestepped by prior administrations, is another ingredient of a package, that for me, kindles the mystery of awe.

Psychologically Sound

Through all of this book I have tried to present President Donald Trump's life as filled with the hopes and fears common to all of us, striving for love, family, success in work, and facing inevitable painful loss and miscalculation. Some events were determined by nature, some by nurture, and some by just plain fate. In this trio of life's determinants, he is recognizably like everyone else. Each of us has foibles of personality, recognizable to those who know us. Many know Trump. Glaring foibles are glaringly broadcast.

Within this usual human picture of Trump are unusual achievements attainable only by a select few in history, but all exist in the presence of a psychologically sound mind. Although I have tried to depict a large range of behaviors in Trump's life, and they are indeed large, none are the result of any mental illness. One must not slip into the thoughtless rationale of condemning political philosophies though psychiatric sleight-of-hand.

The world is awash in amazingly different cultures, languages, and politics. Battles between differing nations are basically political not psychiatric. American intra-national battles are similarly political not psychiatric, engaging one's psychology in the process does not warrant a psychiatric diagnosis. Ultimately, we depend on those remarkable revolutionary framers of our government who "prescribed" votes not diagnoses to settle differences and maintain our national health.

Insufficient Awe

The judgment of history does not rest on the partisan politics of the past. Present day partisan politics is usually determined by local politics—as former Speaker of the House of Representatives Tip O'Neil (D-MA) often remarked, "All politics is local." And being local, partisan politics fade into historical woodwork. President James Polk was reviled in his time and for fifty years after; today his accomplishments are lauded, and his presidency ranked among the greatest. President Harry Truman entered office in 1948 and left office in January 1953 with an approval rating of 31 percent. Upon leaving office the former President Truman and his wife, Bess, drove away from the White House in his old car, all the way to Missouri devoid of secret service escort. In recent decades Truman consistently ranks among the top ten greatest presidents.

Trump is not sprung totally de novo from the American political soil. He was voted in, and represents a momentum of political checks and balances, a swing of the governmental pendulum, which now backs off from internationalism to nationalism. The vast and complex issues emanating from these two tendencies stamps our national character, and will forever be a continuing national dialectic.

Trump's manner of managing change in the balance between internationalism and nationalism while uniquely idiosyncratic is at the same time uniquely democratic. How nature, nurture, and fate, can shape one person to be the vehicle of effective change for many millions is discussable, but remains a mystery, which brings us to awe. Awe, not just for President Trump, but also for the perspicacious framers of our constitution who so long ago crafted our ever-evolving civil bible, and awe for the people of our nation who continue to miraculously struggle with and shape those ideals.

For many, the slings and arrows of today's oppositional media blur the awesome nature of Trump's lifetime achievements along with his historic campaign and his current role in coalescing momentous, national changes. The mind of President Trump is psychologically sound; whether that soundness is matched by his policies is ultimately judged by history.

ACKNOWLEDGMENTS

I am grateful to my family, especially my wife, Cora, and our three sons and their families who, beyond encouragement, have offered thought-provoking ideas through the conception and writing of this book. A special appreciation goes to Dr. Jerrold M. Post with whom I was privileged to spend many hours of germinating discussion about President Trump and from which I then felt compelled to amplify my thoughts in a book. A particular thank you to my literary agent, Scott Mendel, whose skill and intelligence shaped the initial presentation of this book and who was an indispensable guide in the world of publishing. Kudos to David S. Bernstein, Associate Publisher of Bombardier Books, for his grasp of this book's value and enthusiastic endorsement. And much gratitude to Heather King, the managing editor of Post Hill Press, whose skill and unflappable nature monitored the development of the final product. Copyediting is a tough task and appreciative thanks to Matthew Palumbo and Rebecca Stephens for their hard work. In a special twist, allow me to thank all the authors found in my list of references. This book is possible only with the knowledge they have offered all of us.

REFERENCES

Abbott, Bud and Lou Costello. "The Niagara Falls Sketch: Slowly I Turned." youtube.com, Video file, August 24, 2012. https://www.youtube.com/watch?v=8KpsUlvzbkk.

Adams, Scott. "Scott Adams talks about Trump's speech and talking about yourself in the third person." youtube.com, Open Mind, December 10, 2017. [Unfortunately, this video is no longer available.]

Adams, Scott and Dave Rubin. "Trumps Persuasion and Presidency (Full Interview)." youtube.com, November 24, 2017. https://www.youtube.com/watch?v=1WA5pOmSDgQ.

Adams, Scott. *Win Bigly: Persuasion in a World Where Facts Don't Matter.* New York: Penguin Random House, 2017.

Allen, Henry. "Two Partisans Of the Past: Into the '80s." *The Washington Post*, October 8, 1981. https://www.washingtonpost.com/archive/lifestyle/1981/10/08/two-partisans-of-the-past-into-the-80s/3355fe68-fb04-4209-94bf-1e839dc4a03a/.

Alexander, Dan. "After Promising Not To Talk Business With Father, Eric Trump Says He'll Give Him Financial Reports." *Forbes,* March 24, 2017. https://www.forbes.com/sites/

danalexander/2017/03/24/after-promising-not-donald-talk-business-with-father-eric-trump-says-president-give-him-financial-reports/#58eb0fd7359a.

Altman, Alex. "Donald Trump's Suite of Power: Conflicts of Interest in Washington, D.C." *TIME*, June 8, 2017. https://time.com/magazine/us/4810463/june-19th-2017-vol-189-no-23-u-s/.

Arends, Brett. "Morning Movers: Dow Soars as Trump Telegraphs Payrolls Surprise; Costco Slides." *Barron's,* June 1, 2018. https://www.barrons.com/articles/morning-movers-dow-soars-as-trump-telegraphs-payrolls-surprise-costco-slides-1527859273.

Associated Press. "President Trump gains weight, now considered obese." *The Boston Globe*, February 14, 2019. https://www.bostonglobe.com/news/nation/2019/02/14/president-trump-gains-weight-now-considered-obese/Iuwb83rfz4FvlCnXuxg2QP/story.html.

Baker, Peter. "How Trump Has Reshaped the Presidency, and How It's Changed Him, Too." *The New York Times*, April 29, 2017. https://www.nytimes.com/2017/04/29/us/politics/trump-presidency-100-days.html.

Baker, Peter. "Riding an Untamed Horse: Priebus Opens Up on Serving Trump." *The New York Times*, February 14, 2018. https://www.nytimes.com/2018/02/14/us/politics/riding-an-untamed-horse-priebus-opens-up-on-serving-trump.html.

Baker, Peter. "Trump's Contradiction: Assailing 'Left-Wing Mob' as Crowd Chants 'Lock Her Up.'" *The New York Times*,

October 10, 2018. https://www.nytimes.com/2018/10/10/us/politics/trump-rally-opponents.html.

Baker, Peter and Maggie Haberman. "Trump, Defending His Mental Fitness, Says He's a 'Very Stable Genius.'" *The New York Times*, January 6, 2018. https://www.nytimes.com/2018/01/06/us/politics/trump-genius-mental-health.html.

Balingit, Moriah and Danielle Douglas-Gabriel. "Congress rejects much of Betsy DeVos's agenda in spending bill." *The Washington Post*, March 24, 2018. https://www.washingtonpost.com/news/education/wp/2018/03/21/congress-rejects-much-of-betsy-devoss-agenda-in-spending-bill/.

Barron, James. "Overlooked Influences on Donald Trump: A Famous Minister and His Church." *The New York Times*, September 5, 2016. https://www.nytimes.com/2016/09/06/nyregion/donald-trump-marble-collegiate-church-norman-vincent-peale.html.

Barstow, David, Susanne Craig, and Russ Buettner. "Trump Engaged in Suspect Tax Schemes as He Reaped Riches From His Father." *The New York Times*, October 2, 2018. https://www.nytimes.com/interactive/2018/10/02/us/politics/donald-trump-tax-schemes-fred-trump.html.

Bates, Daniel. "Donald Trump pictured in uniform as a cadet captain - before he dodged the Vietnam draft with four deferments and a 'bone spur.'" *Daily Mail*, July 20, 2015. https://www.dailymail.co.uk/news/article-3168648/Donald-Trump-pictured-uniform-cadet-captain-dodged-Vietnam-draft-four-deferments-bone-spur.html.

Begley, Sharon. "'Crazy like a fox': Mental health experts try to get inside Trump's mind." *STAT*, January 30, 2017. https://www.statnews.com/2017/01/30/trump-mental-health/.

Bennhold, Katrin. "A Girl's Killing Shakes Germany's Migration Debate." *The New York Times*, June 8, 2018. https://www.nytimes.com/2018/06/08/world/europe/germany-susanna-murder-migration.html.

Bennhold, Katrin and Melissa Eddy. "Merkel, to Survive, Agrees to Border Camps for Migrants." *The New York Times*, July 2, 2018. https://www.nytimes.com/2018/07/02/world/europe/angela-merkel-migration-coalition.html.

Bennhold, Katrin. "Chemnitz Protests Show New Strength of Germany's Far Right." *The New York Times*, August 30, 2018. https://www.nytimes.com/2018/08/30/world/europe/germany-neo-nazi-protests-chemnitz.html.

Blitzer, Jonathan. "How the D.H.S. Secretary, Kirstjen Nielsen, Became One of President Trump's Fiercest Loyalists." *The New Yorker*, March 1, 2018. https://www.newyorker.com/news/news-desk/how-dhs-secretary-kirstjen-nielsen-became-one-of-president-trumps-fiercest-loyalists.

Borchers, Callum. "Do Trump's alleged affairs even matter?" *The Washington Post*, February 17, 2018. https://www.washingtonpost.com/news/the-fix/wp/2018/02/17/do-trumps-alleged-affairs-even-matter/.

Boyes, Roger. "Muslim migrants behind rise in antisemitism." *The Times*, December 20, 2017. https://www.thetimes.co.uk/article/muslim-migrants-behind-rise-in-antisemitism-rxdsjx2vt.

Boyle, Matthew. "Clinton Cash: Khizr Khan's Deep Legal Financial Connections to Saudi Arabia, Hillary's Clinton Foundation Tie Terror, Immigration, Email Scandals Together." *Breitbart*, August 1, 2016. https://www.breitbart.com/politics/2016/08/01/clinton-cash-khizr-khans-deep-legal-financial-connections-saudi-arabia-hillarys-clinton-foundation-connect-terror-immigration-email-scandals/.

Braslow, M.D., Ph.D., Joel T. and Luke Messac, M.D., Ph.D. "Medicalization and Demedicalization – A Gravely Disabled Homeless Man with Psychiatric Illness." *New England Journal of Medicine* 379 (2018):1885–1888. Accessed September 3, 2019, doi:10.1056/NEJMp1811623. https://www.nejm.org/doi/full/10.1056/NEJMp1811623.

Brenner, Marie. "How Donald Trump and Roy Cohn's Ruthless Symbiosis Changed America." *Vanity Fair*, June 28, 2017. https://www.vanityfair.com/news/2017/06/donald-trump-roy-cohn-relationship.

Burke, Minyvonne. "Good deals run in the family! President Trump's older sister Maryanne, 80, puts her eight-bedroom beachfront Mar-a-Lago mansion on the market for $23 MILLION - more than twice what she paid for it." *Daily Mail*, March 25, 2018. https://www.dailymail.co.uk/news/article-5541163/President-Trumps-older-sister-selling-eight-bedroom-beachfront-home-Florida-23M.html.

Burns, James MacGregor. "James MacGregor Burns." *Wikipedia,* Accessed September 3, 2019. https://en.wikipedia.org/wiki/James_MacGregor_Burns.

Canfield, David. "Donald Trump Once Did a Surprisingly Introspective Interview with Errol Morris about *Citizen*

Kane." *Slate*, October 25, 2016. https://slate.com/culture/2016/10/watch-this-illuminating-interview-between-errol-morris-and-donald-trump-about-citizen-kane.html.

Cassidy, John. "Jared Kushner's Conflicts of Interest Reach a Crisis Point." *The New Yorker*, March 2, 2018. https://www.newyorker.com/news/our-columnists/jared-kushners-conflicts-of-interest-reach-a-crisis-point.

Cassidy, John. "The Entitled Hypocrisy of Ivanka Trump's Personal E-Mail Account." *The New Yorker*, November 20, 2018. https://www.newyorker.com/news/our-columnists/the-entitled-hypocrisy-of-ivanka-trumps-personal-e-mail-account.

Cat, Laura. "Dutch politician commits suicide after revealing she was 'gang raped by Muslims.'" *Voice of Europe*, August 10, 2018. https://voiceofeurope.com/2018/08/dutch-politician-commits-suicide-after-revealing-she-was-gang-raped-by-muslims/.

Cernovich, Mike. "Donald Trump and the War on Free Speech | Mike Cernovich | POLITICS | Rubin Report." YouTube.com, Video File. March 18, 2016. https://www.youtube.com/watch?v=K03gRy6qjKY.

Clement, Scott and Dan Balz. "Americans give Trump negative marks for Helsinki performance, poll finds." *The Washington Post*, July 22, 2018. https://www.washingtonpost.com/politics/americans-give-trump-negative-marks-for-helsinki-performance/2018/07/22/832ec2be-8d19-11e8-a345-a1bf7847b375_story.html.

Cochran, Emilie. "Gallup: Majority of Americans Call Trump Intelligent, Strong and Decisive Leader." *CNSNews*, June 25, 2018. https://www.cnsnews.com/blog/craig-bannister/gallup-majority-americans-call-trump-intelligent-strong-and-decisive-leader.

Colvin, Jill. "'Tremendous victory': Trump celebrates Kavanaugh win." *Yahoo!*, October 7, 2018. https://www.yahoo.com/news/awaiting-kavanaugh-vote-trump-sets-campaign-focus-kansas-163118219--politics.html.

Coulter, Ann. "This Election Will Determine The Survival of Western Civilization." realclearpolitics.com, October 6, 2016. https://www.realclearpolitics.com/video/2016/10/06/ann_coulter_this_election_will_determine_the_survival_of_western_civilization.html.

Cowley, Stacy. "Borrowers Face Hazy Path as Program to Forgive Student Loans Stalls Under Betsy DeVos." *The New York Times*, November 11, 2018. https://www.nytimes.com/2018/11/11/business/student-loans-betsy-devos.html.

Davenport, Coral, Lisa Friedman, and Maggie Haberman. "E.P.A. Chief Scott Pruitt Resigns Under a Cloud of Ethics Scandals." *The New York Times*, July 5, 2018. https://www.nytimes.com/2018/07/05/climate/scott-pruitt-epa-trump.html.

Dawsey, Josh, and Ashley Parker. "'Everyone signed one': Trump is aggressive in his use of nondisclosure agreements, even in government," *The Washington Post*, August 13, 2018. https://www.washingtonpost.com/politics/everyone-signed-one-trump-is-aggressive-in-his-use-of-nondisclosure-agreements-even-in-government/2018/08/13/9d-0315ba-9f15-11e8-93e3-24d1703d2a7a_story.html.

Death Notice. "Deaths Luerssen, Amy." *The New York Times,* June 28, 2006. https://www.nytimes.com/2006/06/28/classified/paid-notice-deaths-luerssen-amy.html?searchResultPosition=1.

Dershowitz, Alan M., "Don't Diagnose Trump – Respond to Him." *Gatestone Institute*, January 12, 2018. https://www.gatestoneinstitute.org/11741/trump-critics-psychiatric-diagnoses.

Draper, Robert. "The Man Behind the President's Tweets." *The New York Times*, April 16, 2018. https://www.nytimes.com/2018/04/16/magazine/dan-scavino-the-secretary-of-offense.html.

Drucker, Jesse and Nadja Popovich. "Trump Could Save More Than $1 Billion Under His New Tax Plan." *The New York Times*, September 28, 2017. https://www.nytimes.com/interactive/2017/09/28/us/politics/trump-tax-benefit.html.

Drucker, Jesse, Kate Kelly, and Ben Protess. "Kushner's Family Business Received Loans After White House Meetings." *The New York Times*, February 28, 2018. https://www.nytimes.com/2018/02/28/business/jared-kushner-apollo-citigroup-loans.html.

Duke, Selwyn. "Germany's Merkel Finally Admits: No-go Zones Exist." *The New American*, March 3, 2018. https://www.thenewamerican.com/world-news/europe/item/28414-germany-s-merkel-finally-admits-no-go-zones-exist.

Ebeling, Paul. "Remember Khizr Khan's Speech at the DNC, He is Back in the News." *Live Trading News*, August 14, 2016.

https://www.livetradingnews.com/remember-khizr-khans-speech-dnc-back-news-11939.html#.XW6xA1VKhhE.

Editorial Board. "There is no fourth branch of government." *Washington Examiner,* February 19, 2017. https://www.washingtonexaminer.com/there-is-no-fourth-branch-of-government.

Editorial Board. "Intrigue in the House of Trump." *The New York Times*, March 1, 2018. https://www.nytimes.com/2018/03/01/opinion/donald-trump-ivanka-jared-kushner-nepotism.html.

Editorial Board. "Jared Kushner Flames Out." *The New York Times*, March 1, 2018. https://www.nytimes.com/2018/03/01/opinion/jared-kushner-donald-trump-nepotism.html.

Editorial Board. "Ivanka Trump's Brand Building at the White House." *The New York Times*, March 1, 2018. https://www.nytimes.com/2018/03/01/opinion/ivanka-trump-donald-nepotism.html.

Editorial Board. "End the War in Afghanistan: It is time to bring American soldiers back home." *The New York Times*, February 3, 2019. https://www.nytimes.com/2019/02/03/opinion/afghanistan-war.html.

Edwards, Tanya. "Donald Trump was 'thinking about my mother' when he met Queen Elizabeth." *Yahoo! Lifestyle*, July 14, 2018. https://www.yahoo.com/lifestyle/donald-trump-thinking-mother-met-queen-elizabeth-222629366.html.

Eilperin, Juliet, Josh Dawsey, and Lisa Rein. "White House concerned Interior Secretary Ryan Zinke violated Federal Rules." *The Washington Post*, November 1, 2018. https://www.washingtonpost.com/national/health-science/

white-house-concerned-interior-secretary-ryan-zinke-violated-federal-rules/2018/11/01/e5e4d2f4-dddc-11e8-b3f0-62607289efee_story.html.

Evans, Heidi. "Inside Trump's Bitter Battle: Nephew's ailing baby caught in the middle." *New York Daily News*, December 19, 2000. https://www.nydailynews.com/archives/news/trumps-bitter-battle-nephew-ailing-baby-caught-middle-article-1.888562.

Evon, Dan. "So You Think You Know the Real Donald Trump?" *Snopes,* Last modified July 25, 2016, Accessed September 4, 2019. https://www.snopes.com/fact-check/so-you-think-you-know-donald-trump/.

Fagan, Cynthia, R. "The Donald 'Bores' In on Marla." *New York Post*, October 25, 2005. https://nypost.com/2005/10/25/the-donald-bores-in-on-marla/.

Ferguson, Niall. "Trump is breaking all the rules, and that could be great for America." *The Boston Globe*, March 12, 2018. https://www.bostonglobe.com/opinion/2018/03/12/trump-breaking-all-rules-and-that-could-great-for-america/xlotc2ETtBEBCLA5Zxpp8O/story.html.

Feuer, Alan. "For Donald Trump, Friends in Few Places." *The New York Times*, March 11, 2016. https://www.nytimes.com/2016/03/13/nyregion/for-donald-trump-friends-in-few-places.html.

Fisher, Marc and Michael Kranish. "Interview with Donald Trump." *The Washington Post* Archives, April 21, 2016. https://www.washingtonpost.com/graphics/politics/trump-revealed-book-reporting-archive/.

Fisher, Marc and Michael Kranish. "Interview with Donald Trump." *The Washington Post* Archives, June 9, 2016. https://www.washingtonpost.com/graphics/politics/trump-revealed-book-reporting-archive/.

Flegenheimer, Matt. "How Long Can John Kelly Hang On?" *The New York Times Magazine*, February 26, 2018. https://www.nytimes.com/2018/02/26/magazine/how-long-can-john-kelly-hang-on.html.

Fleming-Williams, Mark. "How Tax Reform Will Net the U.S. Big Returns." *Econintersect*, March 24, 2018. http://econintersect.com/pages/contributors/contributor.php?post=201803240551.

Frances, Allen. *Twilight of American Sanity*. New York: HarperCollins, 2017.

Frank, Robert, Howard Lorber, and Douglas Elliman. "Inside Trump's inner circle: Howard Lorber." CNBC, October 5, 2016. https://www.cnbc.com/video/2016/10/05/inside-trumps-inner-circle-howard-lorber.html.

Friedersdorf, Conor. "How an Old-School Gossip Columnist Explains Donald Trump." *The Atlantic*, May 28, 2016. https://www.theatlantic.com/politics/archive/2016/05/gossip-columnist-explains-donald-trump/484595/.

Gaddafi, Muammar. "Islam Will Conquer Europe Without Firing A Shot." youtube.com, 2006. https://www.youtube.com/watch?v=WCGYKSEsYFM.

Geist, William, E. "The Expanding Empire of Donald Trump," *The New York Times Magazine*, April 8, 1984. https://www.nytimes.com/1984/04/08/magazine/the-expanding-empire-of-donald-trump.html.

Geller, Pamela. "France Passes Law Saying Children Can Consent to Sex with Adults." *Geller Report*, August 6, 2018. https://gellerreport.com/2018/08/france-law-adults.html/.

Geller, Pamela. "'Like A Military Operation': Migrants Set Ablaze 100 Cars in Swedish 'No-Go Zones' Arson Jihad." *Geller Report*, August 14, 2018. https://gellerreport.com/2018/08/mass-car-burning-jihad-sweden.html/.

Geller, Pamela. "Sweden: New 'No Go Zone' Police Station Rammed by Car, Attacked by Masked Arsonists." *Geller Report*, August 16, 2018. https://gellerreport.com/2018/08/sweden-zone-car.html/.

Geller, Pamela. "Bloodbath Britain: Quadruple Stabbing, Disembowelment, Crime Hits All-time High, Prosecutions Plunge to All-time Low." *Geller Report*, August 19, 2018. https://gellerreport.com/2018/08/broken-britain.html/.

Geller, Pamela. "Screaming for Help, French Woman Burns to Death in Fire After Firefighters Harassed by French 'Youth' During Rescue." *Geller Report*, August 24, 2018. https://gellerreport.com/2018/08/france-woman-dies-fire.html/.

Gearan, Anne. "Trump's doctor says he is in 'very good health' after exam by 11 specialists." *The Boston Globe*, February 8, 2019. https://www.bostonglobe.com/news/nation/2019/02/08/trump-doctor-says-very-good-health-after-exam-specialists/1jsyc5pXGPvGsh98vaRz8I/story.html.

Gerstein, Josh. "Judge approves $25 million Trump University settlement." *Politico*, March 31, 2017. https://www.politico.com/story/2017/03/trump-university-settlement-approved-gonzalo-curiel-236756.

Gill, Lauren. "Trump Is Giving Staffers Secret Assignments and Telling Aides to Hide Them from John Kelly, According to New Report." *Newsweek*, December 3, 2017. https://www.newsweek.com/trump-telling-staffers-hide-his-assignments-john-kelly-according-new-report-729685.

Glaser, Susan B. "The Man Who Put Andrew Jackson in Trump's Oval Office." *Politico Magazine*, January 22, 2018. https://www.politico.com/magazine/story/2018/01/22/andrew-jackson-donald-trump-216493.

Goel, Vindu and Maria Abi-Habib. "Donald Trump Jr. Retreats From Foreign Policy on India Trip." *The New York Times*, February 23, 2018. https://www.nytimes.com/2018/02/23/world/asia/donald-trump-jr-india-modi.html.

Goodstein, Laurie. "Billy Graham Warned Against Embracing a President. His Son Has Gone Another Way." *The New York Times*, February 26, 2018. https://www.nytimes.com/2018/02/26/us/billy-graham-franklin-graham-trump.html.

Greenstein, Fred I. "The Qualities That Bear on Presidential Performance." *Frontline*, October 12, 2004. https://www.pbs.org/wgbh/pages/frontline/shows/choice2004/leadership/greenstein.html.

Grynbaum, Michael M. "Trump Discusses Claims of 'Fake News,' and Their Impact With New York Times Publisher." *The New York Times*, February 1, 2019. https://www.nytimes.com/2019/02/01/business/media/donald-trump-interview-news-media.html.

Guest Book, The Frank Campbell Funeral Chapel. "Norma S. Foerderer Obituary," Accessed September 4, 2019. http://obits.dignitymemorial.com/dignity-memorial/obituary.aspx?n=Norma-Foerderer&lc=1077&pid=166829057&mid=5658370.

Haberman, Maggie. "He's 'One of Us': The Undying Bond Between the Bible Belt and Trump." *The New York Times*, October 14, 2018. https://www.nytimes.com/2018/10/14/us/politics/trump-southern-voters-campaign-rallies.html.

Haberman, Maggie, Michael S. Schmidt, Adam Goldman, and Annie Karni. "Trump Ordered Officials to Give Jared Kushner a Security Clearance." *The New York Times*, February 28, 2019. https://www.nytimes.com/2019/02/28/us/politics/jared-kushner-security-clearance.html.

Hanson, Victor Davis. "Truman May Have Been the Proto-Trump." *American Greatness*, May 9, 2018. https://www.amgreatness.com/2018/05/09/truman-may-have-been-the-proto-trump/.

Hanson, Victor Davis. *The Case for Trump*. New York: Hachette Book Group, 2019.

Harris, Shane, Carol D. Leonnig, and Josh Dawsey. "Kushner's overseas contacts raise concerns as foreign officials seek leverage." *The Washington Post*, February 27, 2018. https://www.washingtonpost.com/world/national-security/kushners-overseas-contacts-raise-concerns-as-foreign-officials-seek-leverage/2018/02/27/16bbc052-18c3-11e8-942d-16a950029788_story.html.

Harwell, Drew. "Interview with Barbara Res." *The Washington Post* Archives, March 31, 2016. https://www.washingtonpost.com/wp-stat/graphics/politics/trump-archive/docs/barbara-res-with-drew-harwell.pdf.

Heil, Emily. "At a white-tie Gridiron dinner, President Trump tries joking: 'I like chaos.'" *The Washington Post*, March 4, 2018. https://www.washingtonpost.com/news/reliable-source/wp/2018/03/04/at-a-white-tie-media-dinner-president-trump-tries-joking-i-like-chaos/.

Hirschtritt, Matthew E. and Renee L. Binder. "A Reassessment of Blaming Mass Shootings on Mental Illness." *JAMA Psychiatry*, April 2018. https://jamanetwork.com/journals/jamapsychiatry/article-abstract/2673380.

Hohmann, James. "The Daily 202: Trump budget highlights disconnect between populist rhetoric and plutocrat reality." *The Washington Post*, February 13, 2018. https://www.washingtonpost.com/news/powerpost/paloma/daily-202/2018/02/13/daily-202-trump-budget-highlights-disconnect-between-populist-rhetoric-and-plutocrat-reality/5a8261a530fb041c3c7d7838/.

Hohmann, James. "The Daily 202: Hope Hicks's evasiveness highlights how far Trump is pushing the envelope on executive privilege." *The Washington Post*, February 28, 2018. https://www.washingtonpost.com/news/powerpost/paloma/daily-202/2018/02/28/daily-202-hope-hicks-s-evasiveness-highlights-how-far-trump-is-pushing-the-envelope-on-executive-privilege/5a960e9530fb047655a069a5/.

Hohmann, James. "The Daily 202: Trump voters stay loyal because they feel disrespected." *The Washington Post*, May 14, 2018. https://www.washingtonpost.com/news/powerpost/paloma/daily-202/2018/05/14/daily-202-trump-voters-stay-loyal-because-they-feel-disrespected/5af8aac530f-b0425887994cc/.

Horowitz, Jason. "Familiar Talk on Women, From an Unfamiliar Trump." *The New York Times*, August 18, 2015. https://www.nytimes.com/2015/08/19/us/politics/familiar-talk-women-from-donald-trump-sister.html.

Horowitz, Jason. "Fred Trump Taught His Son the Essentials of Showboating Self-Promotion." *The New York Times*, August 12, 2016. https://www.nytimes.com/2016/08/13/us/politics/fred-donald-trump-father.html.

Horowitz, Jason. "Back Channel to Trump: Loyal Aide in Trump Tower Acts as Gatekeeper." *The New York Times*, March 27, 2017. https://www.nytimes.com/2017/03/27/us/rhona-graff-donald-trump.html.

Hurd, Dale. "Europe Anti-Semitism Triggers Record Jewish Exodus." CBN News, March 19, 2015. https://www1.cbn.com/cbnnews/world/2015/March/Europe-Anti-Semitism-Triggers-Record-Jewish-Exodus.

Hurt III, Harry. *Lost Tycoon: The Many Lives of Donald J. Trump*. New York: Echo Point Books & Media, 1993.

Inskeep, Steve. "Donald Trump and the Legacy of Andrew Jackson." *The Atlantic*, November 30, 2016. https://www.theatlantic.com/politics/archive/2016/11/trump-and-andrew-jackson/508973/.

Isidore, Chris. "JPMorgan's Jaimie Dimon: I'd love to be president, but…." CNN Business, September 12, 2016. https://money.cnn.com/2016/09/12/news/companies/jamie-dimon-president/index.html.

Italie, Hillel. "Does Trump read? If so, what? Fiery 2005 letter shines light on his relationship with books." *Chicago Tribune*, February 15, 2018. https://www.chicagotribune.com/entertainment/books/ct-trump-letter-literature-20180215-story.html.

Jackson, David. "Donald Trump has treated Kavanaugh accuser Christine Blasey Ford like a Faberge egg, Kellyanne Conway says." *USA Today*, October 3, 2018. https://www.usatoday.com/story/news/politics/2018/10/03/kavanaugh-accuser-christine-ford-treated-like-faberge-egg-conway-says/1509135002/.

Jaffe, Harry. "Who Are Donald Trump's Closest Friends?" *Town & Country*, April 18, 2017. https://www.townandcountrymag.com/society/politics/a9521926/donald-trump-friends/.

Johannsen, Robert W. "Who is James K. Polk? The Enigma of our Eleventh President." *Rutherford B. Hayes Presidential Library & Museums*, February 14, 1999. https://www.rbhayes.org/hayes/who-is-james-k.-polk-the-enigma-of-our-eleventh-president/.

Johnston, David Cay. *The Making of Donald J. Trump*. Brooklyn: Melville House, 2016.

Jung, C. G. *Dreams, Memories, Reflections*. New York: Pantheon, 1961.

Kapadia, Reshma. "The Cold War in Tech Is Real and Investors Can't Ignore It." *Barron's*, February 22, 2019. https://www.barrons.com/articles/the-cold-war-in-tech-is-real-and-investors-cant-ignore-it-51550883601.

Karl, Jonathan, Cecilia Vega, and John Santucci. "Sources: Chief of Staff John Kelly expressed to President Trump willingness to resign." *ABC News*, February 9, 2018. https://abcnews.go.com/Politics/sources-chief-staff-john-kelly-expressed-president-trump/story?id=52970133&yptr=yahoo.

Karni, Annie. "Washington's growing obsession: The 25th Amendment." *Politico*, January 3, 2018. https://www.politico.com/story/2018/01/03/trump-25th-amendment-mental-health-322625.

Katz, Matt. "Trump's Sister, The Judge: A Life Vastly Different, But Often Intertwined." *New Jersey Public Radio*, May 18, 2016. https://www.wqxr.org/story/trumps-sister-judge-life-vastly-different-often-intertwined/.

Kern, Soeren. "Germany: Surge in Migrant Attacks on Police." Gatestone Institute, November 29, 2017. https://www.gatestoneinstitute.org/11459/germany-migrants-attack-police.

Kern, Soeren. "Europe's Migrant Crisis: Millions Still to Come." Gatestone Institute, December 3, 2017. https://www.gatestoneinstitute.org/11480/europe-migrant-crisis-exodus.

Kern, Soeren. "Germany's Migrant Rape Crisis: 'Failure of the State.'" Gatestone Institute, June 11, 2018. https://www.gatestoneinstitute.org/12494/germany-migrants-rape-feldman.

Kern, Soeren. "A Month of Islam and Multiculturism in Britain: June 2018." Gatestone Institute, July 14, 2018. https://www.gatestoneinstitute.org/12695/islam-multiculturalism-britain-june.

Kern, Soeren. "A Month of Multiculturism in Britain: July 2018." Gatestone Institute, August 23, 2018. https://www.gatestoneinstitute.org/12906/multiculturalism-britain-july.

Kern, Soeren. "Italy and Hungary Create 'Anti-Immigration Axis.'" Gatestone Institute, September 1, 2018. https://

www.gatestoneinstitute.org/12945/italy-hungary-immigration.

Kernell, Samuel. *Going Public: New Strategies of Presidential Leadership*, 4th Edition. Washington, D.C.: CQ Press, 2006.

Kerns, Jen. "New polling proves President Trump is right—'Americans are #Dreamers, too.'" *The Hill*, February 3, 2018. https://thehill.com/opinion/white-house/372152-new-polling-proves-president-trump-is-right-americans-are-dreamers-too.

Kerwick, Jack. "The Non Sequitur of Khazir Khan." *Townhall*, August 2, 2016. https://townhall.com/columnists/jack-kerwick/2016/08/02/the-non-sequitur-of-khazir-khan-n2201162.

Kessler, Glenn. "2,140 false or misleading claims attributed to Trump in first year." *The Boston Globe*, January 22, 2018. https://www3.bostonglobe.com/news/nation/2018/01/21/false-misleading-claims-attributed-trump-first-year/CmrceAadHJalEaWmStp9xO/story.html?camp=bg%3Abrief%3Arss%3Afeedly&rss_id=feedly_rss_brief&s_campaign=bostonglobe%3Asocialflow%3Atwitter&arc404=true.

Kessler, Glenn, Rizzo, Salvador, Kelly, Meg, "President Trump has made over 5,000 false or misleading claims." *The Washington Post*, September 13, 2018. https://beta.washingtonpost.com/politics/2018/09/13/president-trump-has-made-more-than-false-or-misleading-claims/.

Kessler, Glenn, Salvador Rizzo, and Meg Kelly. "Fact-checking President Trump's 2019 State of the Union address." *The Washington Post*, February 6, 2019. https://www.washingtonpost.com/politics/2019/02/06/fact-checking-president-trumps-state-union-address/.

Kessler, Ronald. "The two Donald Trumps." *The Washington Times*, August 3, 2015. https://www.washingtontimes.com/news/2015/aug/3/ronald-kessler-the-two-donald-trumps/.

Kim, Seung Min and Josh Dawsey. "'He just picks up': Trump and the lawmakers he loves to talk to on the phone." *The Washington Post*, February 19, 2019. https://www.washingtonpost.com/politics/he-just-picks-up-trump-and-the-lawmakers-he-loves-to-talk-to-on-the-phone/2019/02/18/f7b846b4-3075-11e9-ac6c-14eea99d5e24_story.html.

King, Ruth S. "Victor Davis Hanson: 'The Case for Trump.'" *Ruthfully Yours*, March 2, 2019. http://www.ruthfullyyours.com/2019/03/01/victor-davis-hanson-the-case-for-trump/.

King, Ruth. "*The New York Times*' Fact-Check Fail the *NYT*'s 'fact-checking' article on Trump's SOTU address deserves special ridicule." *Ruthfully Yours*, February 2, 2018. http://www.ruthfullyyours.com/?s=The+New+York+Times%E2%80%99+Fact-Check+Fail+the+NYT%E2%80%99s+%E2%80%9Cfact-checking%E2%80%9D+article+on+Trump%E2%80%99s+SOTU+address+deserves+special+ridicule.

Kinzer, Stephen. "Three heretic authors take on the US foreign-policy blob." *The Boston Globe*, November 23, 2018. https://www.bostonglobe.com/opinion/2018/11/23/three-heretic-authors-take-foreign-policy-blob/DjZFYl4Glfmmwz9G5rwnyI/story.html.

Klein, Christopher. "10 Things You May Not Know About Andrew Jackson." *History*, March 15, 2017. https://www.history.com/news/10-things-you-may-not-know-about-andrew-jackson.

Klein, Rebecca. "DeVos Finally Agrees Federal Dollars Shouldn't Fund LGBTQ Discrimination in Schools." *HuffPost*, March 20, 2018. https://www.huffpost.com/entry/devos-lgbtq-discrimination-private-schools_n_5ab14474e4b054d118dd7cc8.

Klemesrud, Judy. "Donald Trump, Real Estate Promoter, Builds Image as He Buys Buildings." *The New York Times*, November 1, 1976. https://www.nytimes.com/1976/11/01/archives/donald-trump-real-estate-promoter-builds-image-as-he-buys-buildings.html.

Koffler, Keith. "North Korea's nuclear ambitions met their match in President Donald Trump."*ABC News*, April 27, 2018. https://www.nbcnews.com/think/opinion/north-korea-s-nuclear-ambitions-met-their-match-president-donald-ncna868831.

Kranish, Michael. "'He's better than this,' says Thomas Barrack, Trump's loyal whisperer." *The Washington Post*, October 11, 2017. https://www.washingtonpost.com/politics/hes-better-than-this-says-thomas-barrack-trumps-loyal-whisperer/2017/10/10/067fc776-a215-11e7-8cfe-d5b912fabc99_story.html.

Kranish, Michael. "How the relationship between Trump and Bloomberg went into a tailspin." *The Washington Post*, January 31, 2019. https://www.washingtonpost.com/politics/how-the-relationship-between-trump-and-bloomberg-went-into-a-tailspin/2019/01/31/95ee0914-1ff9-11e9-9145-3f74070bbdb9_story.html.

Kranish, Michael and Marc Fisher. *Trump Revealed.* New York: Simon and Schuster, 2016.

Kruse, Michael. "The Mystery of Mary Trump." *Politico Magazine*, November/December, 2017. https://www.politico.com/magazine/story/2017/11/03/mary-macleod-trump-donald-trump-mother-biography-mom-immigrant-scotland-215779.

Landler, Mark and Maggie Haberman. "Trump's Chaos Theory for the Oval Office Is Taking Its Toll." *The New York Times*, March 1, 2018. https://www.nytimes.com/2018/03/01/us/politics/trump-chaos-oval-office.html.

Landler, Mark, Maggie Haberman, and Harris Gardiner. "In Replacing Tillerson With Pompeo, Trump Turns to Loyalists Who Reflect 'America First' Views." *The New York Times*, March 13, 2018. https://www.nytimes.com/2018/03/13/us/politics/trump-tillerson-pompeo-america-first.html.

Laughland, Oliver. "Ex-Trump workers describe egocentric micromanager: 'Donald loves Donald.'" *The Guardian*, March 14, 2016. https://www.theguardian.com/us-news/2016/mar/14/donald-trump-former-employee-interviews-ego-diversity.

Leach, Katie. "New York Times photographer: Trump gives us more access than Obama." *Washington Examiner*, February 9, 2018. https://www.washingtonexaminer.com/new-york-times-photographer-trump-gives-us-more-access-than-obama.

Leibovich, Mark. "How Lindsey Graham Went From Trump Skeptic to Trump Sidekick." *The New York Times Magazine*, February 25, 2019. https://www.nytimes.com/2019/02/25/magazine/lindsey-graham-what-happened-trump.html.

Lee, Bandy X. *The Dangerous Case of Donald Trump: 27 Psychiatrists and Mental Health Experts Assess a President.* New York: St. Martin's Press, 2017.

Leonhardt, David and Prasad Philbrick. "Trump's Corruption: The Definitive List." *The New York Times*, October 28, 2018. https://www.nytimes.com/2018/10/28/opinion/trump-administration-corruption-conflicts.html.

Leonnig, Carol D., Shane Harris, and Greg Jaffe. "Breaking with tradition, Trump skips president's written intelligence report and relies on oral briefings." *The Washington Post*, February 9, 2018. https://www.washingtonpost.com/politics/breaking-with-tradition-trump-skips-presidents-written-intelligence-report-for-oral-briefings/2018/02/09/b7ba569e-0c52-11e8-95a5-c396801049ef_story.html.

Lewandowski, Corey R. and David N. Bossie. *Let Trump Be Trump* New York: Hachette Book Group, 2017.

Linskey, Annie. "Inside the Trump Tweet Machine: Staff-written posts, bad grammar (on purpose), and delight in the chaos." *The Boston Globe*, May 22, 2018. https://www3.bostonglobe.com/news/nation/2018/05/21/trump-tweets-include-grammatical-errors-and-some-them-are-purpose/JeL7AtKLPevJDIIOMG7TrN/story.html?arc404=true.

Lorber, Howard and Douglas Elliman. "Inside the Trump White House: Howard Lorber." CNBC, November 14, 2016.

https://www.cnbc.com/video/2016/11/14/inside-the-trump-white-house-howard-lorber.html.

Luce, Edward. "Henry Kissinger: 'We are in a very, very grave period.'" *Financial Times*, July 20, 2018. https://www.ft.com/content/926a66b0-8b49-11e8-bf9e-8771d5404543.

Lybrand, Holmes, et.al. "Fact-checking Trump's speech declaring a national emergency." CNN, February 17, 2019. https://www.cnn.com/2019/02/15/politics/fact-check-trump-national-emergency-immigration-speech/index.html.

Madani, Doha. "Betsy DeVos Gets Hammered For Shielding Student Loan Servicers From State Regs." *HuffPost*, March 20, 2018. https://www.huffpost.com/entry/betsy-devos-rosa-delauro-student-loans_n_5ab15a0de4b008c9e5f21760.

Mahler, Jonathan and Matt Flegenheimer. "What Donald Trump Learned From Joseph McCarthy's Right-Hand Man." *The New York Times*, June 20, 2016. https://www.nytimes.com/2016/06/21/us/politics/donald-trump-roy-cohn.html.

Mathis-Lilley, Ben. "Longtime Trump Adviser Claims Khizr Khan Is a Terrorist Agent." *Slate*, August 1, 2016. https://slate.com/news-and-politics/2016/08/roger-stone-says-khizr-khan-is-a-muslim-brotherhood-saboteur.html.

McCarthy, Andrew C. "Islam and the Jihad in London." *National Review*, March 25, 2017. https://www.nationalreview.com/2017/03/westminster-attack-khalid-masood-islamic-europe-mosques-no-go-zones/.

Meotti, Giulio. “Belgium: First Islamic State in Europe?” Gatestone Institute, April 22, 2018. https://www.gatestoneinstitute.org/12203/belgium-islamic-state.

Meotti, Giulio. “Europe: Prayer in Public Spaces.” Gatestone Institute, August 11, 2018. https://www.gatestoneinstitute.org/12568/europe-public-prayer.

Montalbano, Ginny. “Despite Hollywood’s Scorn, Melania Trump Has Accomplished Much as First Lady.” *The Daily Signal*, January 24, 2018. https://www.dailysignal.com/2018/01/24/despite-hollywoods-scorn-melania-trump-has-accomplished-much-as-first-lady/.

Mosconi, Angela. “Fred Trump, Dad of Donald, Dies At 93.” *New York Post*, June 26, 1999. https://nypost.com/1999/06/26/fred-trump-dad-of-donald-dies-at-93/.

Neustadt, Richard E. *Presidential Power and the Modern Presidents: The Politics of Leadership from Roosevelt to Reagan.* New York: The Free Press/Simon & Schuster, 1990.

Noack, Rick. “Another top official says Trump deserves a Nobel Peace Prize (unless he messes things up.” *The Washington Post*, May 8, 2018. https://www.washingtonpost.com/news/world/wp/2018/05/08/another-top-official-says-trump-deserves-a-nobel-peace-prize-unless-he-messes-things-up/.

Nuzzi, Olivia. “What Hope Hicks Knows.” *New York Magazine*, March 18, 2018. http://nymag.com/intelligencer/2018/03/what-hope-hicks-learned-in-washington.html.

O’Connell, Jonathan, David A. Fahrenthold, and Jack Gillum. “As the ‘King of Debt,’ Trump borrowed to build his empire. Then he began spending hundreds of millions in cash." *The Washington Post*, May 5, 2018. https://www.washingtonpost.com/politics/as-the-king-of-debt-trump-borrowed-to-build-his-empire-then-he-began-spending-hundreds-of-millions-in-cash/2018/05/05/28fe54b4-44c4-11e8-8569-26fda6b404c7_story.html.

Odumeru, James A. and Ifeanyi George Ogbonna. "Transformational vs. Transactional Leadership Theories: Evidence in Literature." *International Review of Management and Business Research 2,* no. 2 (2013): 355-361, http://www.irmbrjournal.com/papers/1371451049.pdf.

Osnos, Evan. "Three Key Questions About Donald Trump's Summit with Kim Jong Un." *The New Yorker*, March 9, 2018. https://www.newyorker.com/news/daily-comment/three-key-questions-about-donald-trumps-summit-with-kim-jong-un.

Parton, James. *Life of Andrew Jackson Volume One*." New York: Mason Brothers, 1861.

Peale, Norman Vincent. *The Power of Positive Thinking*. New York: Touchstone/Simon & Schuster, 1952.

Peebles, Maurice and Keane Macadaeg. "9 Things You Didn't Know About Donald Trump's Baseball Career." *Complex*, November 2, 2016. https://www.complex.com/sports/2016/11/donald-trump-baseball/.

Peretz, Evgenia. "Inside The Trump Marriage: Melania's Burden." *Vanity Fair*, April 21, 2017. https://www.vanityfair.com/news/2017/04/donald-melania-trump-marriage.

Peters, Jeremy W. "Trump's New Judicial Litmus Test: Shrinking 'the Administrative State.'" *The New York Times*, March

26, 2018. https://www.nytimes.com/2018/03/26/us/politics/trump-judges-courts-administrative-state.html.

Pirro, Jeanine. *Liars, Leakers, and Liberals: The Case Against the Anti-Trump Conspiracy*. New York: Hachette Book Group, 2018.

Post, Jerrold M. *Narcissism and Politics: Dreams of Glory*. New York: Cambridge University Press, 2015.

Pour, Nima Gholam Ali. "Sweden's Government Funds Anti-Semitism." Gatestone Institute, August 10, 2018. https://www.gatestoneinstitute.org/12814/sweden-antisemitism.

Reeves, Richard. "What is 'presidential greatness'?" CNN, October 28, 2012. https://www.cnn.com/2012/10/28/opinion/opinion-presidential-greatness/index.html.

Resnick, Brian. "Psychiatry's 'Goldwater Rule' has never met a test like Donald Trump." *Vox*, May 25, 2017. https://www.vox.com/science-and-health/2017/5/25/15680354/psychiatry-goldwater-rule-trump.

Riotta, Chris. "Jared Kushner Can't Pass His Security Clearance Investigation, Officials Say." *Newsweek*, December 1, 2017. https://www.newsweek.com/jared-kushner-security-clearance-white-house-access-ivanka-donald-trump-723993.

Roberts, Roxanne. "Washington society and Team Trump: A year in, the fear and loathing is mutual." *The Washington Post*, February 26, 2018. https://www.washingtonpost.com/lifestyle/style/washington-society-and-team-trump-a-year-in-the-fear-and-loathing-is-mutual/2018/02/26/3767184a-1299-11e8-9065-e55346f6de81_story.html.

Rogers, Katie. "Does Melania Trump Ever Tell the President to Put Away His Phone? 'Yes!'" *The New York Times*, October

6, 2018. https://www.nytimes.com/2018/10/06/world/africa/melania-trump-africa-trip-egypt.html.

Rogers, Katie, Julie Hirschfeld Davis, and Maggie Haberman. "Melania Trump, a Mysterious First Lady, Weathers a Chaotic White House." *The New York Times*, August 17, 2018. https://www.nytimes.com/2018/08/17/us/politics/melania-trump-first-lady.html.

Rose, Charlie. "Interview with Donald Trump." *Charlie Rose*, November 6, 1992. https://charlierose.com/videos/14730.

Roth, Sheldon. *Psychotherapy: The Art of Wooing Nature*. New Jersey: Jason Aronson, Inc, 1987.

Rozhon, Tracie. "Fred C. Trump, Postwar Master Builder of Housing for Middle Class, Dies at 93." *The New York Times*, June 26, 1999. https://www.nytimes.com/1999/06/26/nyregion/fred-c-trump-postwar-master-builder-of-housing-for-middle-class-dies-at-93.html.

Rucker, Phillip, Ashley Parker, and Josh Dawsey. "'Jared has faded': Inside the 28 days of tumult that left Kushner badly diminished." *The Washington Post*, March 2, 2018. https://www.washingtonpost.com/politics/jared-has-faded-inside-the-28-days-of-tumult-that-left-kushner-badly-diminished/2018/03/02/62acb9ce-1ca8-11e8-9de1-147dd2df3829_story.html.

Rucker, Phillip, Ashley Parker, and Josh Dawsey. "'Pure madness': Dark days inside the White House as Trump shocks and rages." *The Washington Post*, March 3, 2018. https://www.washingtonpost.com/politics/pure-madness-dark-days-inside-the-white-house-as-trump-shocks-

and-rages/2018/03/03/9849867c-1e72-11e8-9de1-147dd2df3829_story.html.

Rucker, Phillip, Ashley Parker, Sean Sullivan, and Seung Min Kim. "'Willing to go to the mat:' How Trump and Republicans carried Kavanaugh to the cusp of confirmation." *The Washington Post*, October 5, 2018. https://www.washingtonpost.com/politics/willing-to-go-to-the-mat-how-trump-and-republicans-carried-kavanaugh-to-the-cusp-of-confirmation/2018/10/05/7cdf0d0e-c81c-11e8-b1ed-1d2d65b86d0c_story.html.

Salzillio, Leslie. "Can Ben Carson Really Be This Inept and Incompetent?" *AlterNet*, October 30, 2017. https://www.alternet.org/2017/10/ben-carson-doesnt-know-his-own-budget/.

Samuels, Robert and Jenna Johnson. "'It's not my thing': A history of Trump's shifting relationship with the LGBT community." *The Washington Post*, July 26, 2017. https://www.washingtonpost.com/politics/its-not-my-thing-a-history-of-trumps-shifting-relationship-with-the-lgbt-community/2017/07/26/92920302-7220-11e7-8f39-eeb-7d3a2d304_story.html.

Sargent, Greg. "Trump's ugly attacks on Blasey Ford could save the Senate for Republicans. Really." *The Washington Post*, October 8, 2018. https://www.washingtonpost.com/blogs/plum-line/wp/2018/10/08/trumps-ugly-attacks-on-blasey-ford-could-save-the-senate-for-republicans-really/.

Sawyer, Diane. "Diane Sawyer Interviews Donald Trump." *Good Morning America*, December 2, 1999. https://factba.se/

transcript/donald-trump-interview-abc-diane-sawyer-december-2-1999.

Schlesinger, Arthur M., Jr. "Rating the Presidents: Washington to Clinton." *Frontline*, October 12, 2004. https://www.pbs.org/wgbh/pages/frontline/shows/choice2004/leadership/schlesinger.html.

Schoen, W. John. "After 500 days, hundreds of White House jobs remain unfilled by Trump administration." CNBC, June 4, 2018. https://www.cnbc.com/2018/06/04/after-500-days-dozens-of-white-house-jobs-remain-unfilled.html.

Schwartzman, Paul and Miller E. Michael. "Confident. Incorrigible. Bully: Little Donny was a lot like candidate Donald Trump." *The Washington Post*, June 22, 2016. https://www.washingtonpost.com/lifestyle/style/young-donald-trump-military-school/2016/06/22/f0b3b164-317c-11e6-8758-d58e76e11b12_story.html.

Sellers, Frances Stead. "Donald Trump, a champion of women? His female employees think so." *The Washington Post*, November 24, 2015. https://www.washingtonpost.com/politics/donald-trump-a-champion-of-women-his-female-employees-think-so/2015/11/23/7eafac80-88da-11e5-9a07-453018f9a0ec_story.html.

Shapiro, Rebecca. "Elizabeth Warren Tells Ben Carson To His Face: You Should Be Fired." *Huffington Post*, March 22, 2018. https://www.huffpost.com/entry/elizabeth-warren-tells-ben-carson-to-his-face-you-should-be-fired_n_5ab451e9e4b008c9e5f5c427.

Shear, Michael D. and Lawrence K. Altman. "Trump Has Perfect Cognitive Test Score, White House Physician Says." *The New York Times*, January 16, 2018. https://www.nytimes.com/2018/01/16/us/politics/trump-health-exam-doctor-cognitive-test.html.

Shear, Michael D. "Trump Stuns Lawmakers with Seeming Embrace of Comprehensive Gun Control." *The New York Times*, February 28, 2018. https://www.nytimes.com/2018/02/28/us/politics/trump-gun-control.html.

"Short-lived campaign newspaper to elect Andrew Jackson." *Timothy Hughes Rare & Early Newspapers*. Accessed September 4, 2019. http://www.rarenewspapers.com/view/609728.

Shribman, David, M. "What makes a leader great? Sharing lessons from 4 presidents." *The Boston Globe*, September 20, 2018. https://www.bostonglobe.com/arts/books/2018/09/20/what-makes-leader-great/QYpMIWxvoN2b2Xepbo1mkN/story.html.

Sit, Ryan. "Trump Still Hasn't Appointed A U.S. Ambassador To South Korea Or Filled 56 Other Such Vacancies." *Newsweek*, March 8, 2018. https://www.newsweek.com/donald-trump-north-korea-south-korea-no-united-states-ambassador-56-countries-837029.

Smith, Allan. "There's been a mysterious change in Trump's demeanor – and no one knows why." *Business Insider*, February 2, 2018. https://www.businessinsider.com/trump-change-in-demeanor-2018-2.

Smith-Spark, Laura. "Anti-Semitism is so bad in Britain that some Jews are planning to leave." CNN, August 17, 2018.

https://www.cnn.com/2018/08/17/uk/uk-anti-semitism-intl/index.html.

Stephens, Bret. "For Once I Am Grateful for Trump." *The New York Times*, October 4, 2018. https://www.nytimes.com/2018/10/04/opinion/trump-kavanaugh-ford-allegations.html.

Stolberg, Sheryl Gay. "What Happened to Lindsey Graham? He's Become a Conservative 'Rock Star.'" *The New York Times*, November 2, 2018. https://www.nytimes.com/2018/11/02/us/politics/lindsey-graham-trump-midterms.html.

Stracqualursi, Veronica. "Melania Trump says President Trump's alleged affairs are 'not concern and focus of mine.'" CNN, October 12, 2018. https://www.cnn.com/2018/10/12/politics/melania-trump-marriage-president-alleged-affairs/index.html.

Swan, Jonathan. "Scoop: Trump's secret, shrinking schedule." *Axios*, January 7, 2018. https://www.axios.com/scoop-trumps-secret-shrinking-schedule-1515364904-ab76374a-6252-4570-a804-942b3f851840.html.

Tackett, Michael. "Trump Rallies a Florida Crowd in Support of an Alabama Senate Candidate." *The New York Times*, December 8, 2017. https://www.nytimes.com/2017/12/08/us/politics/trump-moore-florida-alabama.html.

Tavani, Shveta. "Things you didn't know about Barron Trump." thebollywoodticket.com, May 20, 2018. http://www.thebollywoodticket.com/2018/01/things-you-didnt-know-about-barron-trump/

The New York Times, "Read Excerpts: The Times Publisher Asks Trump About 'Anti-Press Rhetoric.'" *The New York Times*, February 1, 2019. https://www.nytimes.com/2019/02/01/us/politics/trump-times-publisher-sulzberger-transcript.html.

The Three Stooges. "Slowly I Turned." youtube.com, Video File, April 1, 2012. https://www.youtube.com/watch?v=MYP1OBZfFK0.

Thrush, Glenn. "Ben Carson Defends Buying $31,000 Dining Set to Congress: 'I Left It to My Wife.'" *The New York Times*, March 20, 2018. https://www.nytimes.com/2018/03/20/us/ben-carson-hud-dining-room.html.

Thrush, Glenn. "Under Ben Carson, HUD Scales Back Fair Housing Enforcement." *The New York Times*, March 28, 2018. https://www.nytimes.com/2018/03/28/us/ben-carson-hud-fair-housing-discrimination.html.

Tolentino, Jia. "Ivanka Trump Wrote a Painfully Oblivious Book for Basically No One." *The New Yorker*, May 4, 2017. https://www.newyorker.com/books/page-turner/ivanka-trump-wrote-a-painfully-oblivious-book-for-basically-no-one.

Trump, Donald J. with Tony Schwartz. *The Art of the Deal.* New York: Ballantine Books, 1987.

Trump, Donald J. with Kate Bohner. *The Art of the Comeback.* New York: Times Books/Random House, 1997.

Trump, Donald J. with Dave Shiflett. *The America We Deserve.* Los Angeles: Renaissance Books, 2000.

Trump, Donald J. with Meredith McIver. *How to Get Rich.* New York: Random House, 2004.

Trump, Donald J. with Meredith McIver. *Think Like a Billionaire*. New York: Random House, 2004.

Trump, Donald J. and Bill Zanker. *Think Big and Kick Ass in Business and Life*. New York: HarperCollins, 2007.

Trump, Donald J. with Meredith McIver. *Never Give Up*. Hoboken: John Wiley & Sons, 2008.

Trump, Donald J. *Time to Get Tough: Making America #1 Again*. Washington, D.C.: Regnery Publishing, 2011.

Trump, Donald J. with Robert T. Kiyosaki. *Midas Touch*. Scottsdale: Plata Publishing, 2011.

Trump, Donald J. *Crippled America*. New York: Threshold Editions, 2015.

Trump, Donald J. *Great Again: How to Fix Our Crippled America*. New York: Threshold Editions/Simon and Schuster, 2016.

Trump, Ivana. *Raising Trump*. New York: Gallery Publishing Group/Simon and Schuster, 2017.

u/narf8h1, "President Trump spots his little brother Robert in the crowd...a very nice moment." *Reddit*, July 17, 2018. https://www.reddit.com/r/The_Donald/comments/8z7dn5/president_trump_spots_his_little_brother_robert/.

Vazquez, Joseph. "The Federal Bureaucracy: The Fourth Branch of Government." *Odyssey*, December 12, 2016. https://www.theodysseyonline.com/federal-bureaucracy-fourth-branch-government.

Viser, Matt and Yun Wu. "11 months, 1 president, 2,417 tweets." *The Boston Globe*, December 26, 2017. https://apps.bostonglobe.com/opinion/graphics/2017/12/president-twitter/.

Voice of Europe. "Macron is losing control over Islam-dominated no-go areas in France, asks public for help." *Voice of Europe*, June 11, 2018. https://voiceofeurope.com/2018/06/macron-is-losing-control-over-islam-dominated-no-go-areas-in-france-asks-public-for-help/.

Voice of Europe. "Paris is a mess: Up to 400,000 illegal immigrants live in just one suburb." *Voice of Europe*, July 5, 2018. https://voiceofeurope.com/2018/07/paris-is-a-mess-up-to-400000-illegal-immigrants-live-in-just-one-suburb/.

Wang, Evelyn. "Whether or Not the Trumps Keep Them, Separate Bedrooms Are the Ultimate Status Symbol." *Vanity Fair*, May 31, 2017. https://www.vanityfair.com/style/2017/05/separate-bedrooms-trumps.

Weber, Peter. "White House Chief of Staff John Kelly also apparently wants to know what Jared and Ivanka do all day." *The Week*, March 2, 2018. https://theweek.com/speedreads/758552/white-house-chief-staff-john-kelly-also-apparently-wants-know-what-jared-ivanka-all-day.

Weiland, Noah. "Evangelicals, Having Backed Trump, Find White House 'Front Door is Open.'" *The New York Times*, February 7, 2018. https://www.nytimes.com/2018/02/07/us/politics/trump-evangelicals-national-prayer-breakfast.html.

"What is 'presidential greatness'?" CNN, October 28, 2012. https://www.cnn.com/2012/10/28/opinion/opinion-presidential-greatness/index.html.

Wheeler, Brian. "The Trump era's top-selling dystopian novels." BBC News, January 29, 2017. https://www.bbc.com/news/magazine-38764041.

Winch, Guy. "Study: Half of All Presidents Suffered from Mental Illness." *Psychology Today*, February 2, 2016. https://www.psychologytoday.com/us/blog/the-squeaky-wheel/201602/study-half-all-presidents-suffered-mental-illness.

Winnicott, D. W. *Collected Papers: Through Paediatrics to Psycho-Analysis.* London: Tavistock Publications, Ltd, 1958.

Wolf, Michael. *Fire and Fury: Inside the Trump White House.* New York: Henry Holt and Co, 2018.

Wood, Braelyn. "20 Quotes from Donald & Melania Trump About Love & Marriage." *Cosmopolitan*, January 31, 2017. https://www.cosmopolitan.com/politics/a8646248/donald-and-melania-trump-quotes-about-love-and-marriage/.

Wright, Robin. "With Mike Pompeo at the State Department, Are the Über-Hawks Winning?" *The New Yorker*, March 13, 2018. https://www.newyorker.com/news/news-desk/with-mike-pompeo-at-the-state-department-are-the-uber-hawks-winning.

Yourish, Karen and Denise Lu. "Trump as Optimist, Salesman or Bully: Mixing Messages in His First Year." *The New York Times*, January 31, 2018. https://www.nytimes.com/interactive/2018/01/31/us/politics/many-sides-of-trump.html.

Zadrozny, Brandy. "Donald Trump Made Out With Marla Maples as She Delivered His Child." *The Daily Beast*, September 5, 2016. https://www.thedailybeast.com/donald-trump-made-out-with-marla-maples-as-she-delivered-his-child.

Zak, Dan. "Eric and Don have the Trump name, the money, the genes. Here's what makes them different." *The Washington Post*, May 18, 2016. https://www.washingtonpost.com/

lifestyle/style/trump-raised-sons-who-became-his-emissaries-but-not-the-way-you-might-think/2016/05/18/3ca1c-fa8-faa4-11e5-886f-a037dba38301_story.html.